Caring for the Dying Patient and the Family

Third edition

Edited by

Joy Robbins
Former Senior Tutor at St Joseph's Hospice, London, UK

and

Janet Moscrop
Study Centre Coordinator at St Joseph's Hospice, London, UK

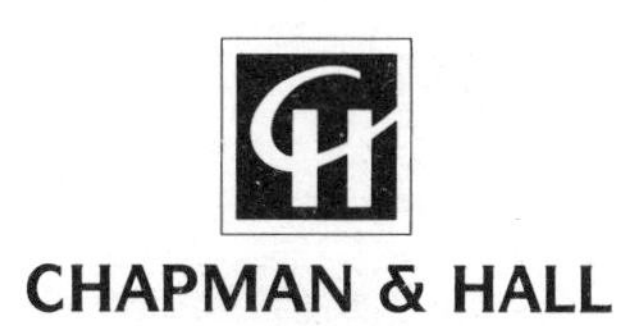

CHAPMAN & HALL
London · Glasgow · Weinheim · New York · Tokyo · Melbourne · Madras

Published by Chapman & Hall, 2–6 Boundary Row, London SE1 8HN, UK

Chapman & Hall, 2–6 Boundary Row, London SE1 8HN, UK

Blackie Academic & Professional, Wester Cleddens Road, Bishopbriggs, Glasgow G64 2NZ, UK

Chapman & Hall GmbH, Pappelallee 3, 69469 Weinheim, Germany

Chapman & Hall USA, One Penn Plaza, 41st Floor, New York NY 10119, USA

Chapman & Hall Japan, ITP-Japan, Kyowa Building, 3F, 2-2-1 Hirakawacho, Chiyoda-ku, Tokyo 102, Japan

Chapman & Hall Australia, Thomas Nelson Australia, 102 Dodds Street, South Melbourne, Victoria 3205, Australia

Chapman & Hall India, R. Seshadri, 32 Second Main Road, CIT East, Madras 600 035, India

Distributed in the USA and Canada by Singular Publishing Group Inc., 4284 41st Street, San Diego, California 92105

First edition 1983
Second edition 1989
Reprinted 1992
Third edition 1995

Typeset in Times Roman 10/12 by Acorn Bookwork, Salisbury, Wiltshire
Printed in Great Britain by Clays Ltd, St Ives PLC

ISBN 0 412 57840 9 1 56593 328 1 (USA)

The use of the terms ‘he’ and ‘his’ is not indicative of a specific gender and should be taken to refer to both men and women throughout.

A catalogue record for this book is available from the British Library

∞ Printed on permanent acid-free text paper, manufactured in accordance with ANSI/NISO Z39.48-1992 and ANSI/NISO Z39.48-1984 (Permanence of Paper).

Contents

Contributors

Karen Baldry, MCSP
Physiotherapist, St Joseph's Hospice, London

Jennifer Clark, BEd (Hons), Dip.Nursing (Lond.), RNT, RCNT, RSCN, RGN, SCM
Nurse Teacher, St Joseph's Hospice, London.

Alison Cotterill, MSCP, SRP
Physiotherapist, Garden House Hospice, Letchworth

Dennis Donald, Anglican Minister and Chaplain
Eden Valley Hospice, Carlisle

Jane Eisenhauer, BA (Hons)
Arts & Media Associate, St Joseph's Hospice, London

Jennifer Ellwood, RGN, SCM
Clinical Nurse Specialist, Palliative Care at Homerton Hospital, London

Elizabeth Faulkner, RGN, SGM, RNT, ALCM, LLCM
Nurse Teacher, Pilgrim's Hospice, Canterbury and Thanet

Sr Jacinta Forde, RSC, RGN
Ward Sister, St Joseph's Hospice, London

Sr Florence Haines, RSC, BA, Higher Dip. Ed.
Voluntary Services Coordinator, St Joseph's Hospice, London

Anthea Hare, SRN, RSCN, RCNT
Founder/Project Director, Richard House "Home from Home", Newham

Dr Louis Heyse-Moore, MBBS, DOBst, RCOG, DCH, MRCGP, MRCP (UK), DM
Medical Director, St Joseph's Hospice, London

Rosemary Hurdman, CQSW
Social Work Coordinator, St Joseph's Hospice, London

Lucinda Langford, RGN, DN
Macmillan Nurse, St Joseph's Hospice, Home Care Team, London

Mary McDermott, RGN, RM
Ward Sister, St Joseph's Hospice, London

Sr Helena McGilly, RCS, RGN, RM, NDN, Cert. Matron
Our Lady's Hospice, Dublin

David Morrell, Chaplain
Rowcroft, Torbay & South Devon Hospice

Janet Moscrop, RGN, Dip.Nursing (Lond.), Cert. Ed., RNT
Study Centre Coordinator, St Joseph's Hospice, London

Janet Nevitt, RGN, RSCN, RCNT, RNT
Day Hospice Organizer, Garden House Hospice, Letchworth

Georgina Nunn, RGN, DN, PH ITEC Dip.
Massage Therapist, Garden House Hospice, Letchworth

Fr Tom O'Connor, OSCam, LPh, BD
Chaplain, St Joseph's Hospice, London

Jacqueline Ougham, SEN
State Enrolled Nurse, Garden House Hospice, Letchworth

Christopher Quinn, RGN
Clinical Nurse Specialist, HIV/AIDS, Southend

Sharon Quinn, RGN
Clinical Nurse Specialist, HIV/AIDS, Basildon & Thurrock

Joan Ramsay, MSC, RGN, RSCN, Dip. Nursing (Lond.), Cert.Ed., RNT
Principal Lecturer, University of Luton

Shirley Richards, CQSW
Social Worker, Bereavement Services, St Joseph's Hospice, London.

Joy Robbins, BA, RGN, SCM, RNT
Bereavement Visitor (formerly Senior Tutor, St Joseph's Hospice, London)

Sr Philomena Sherry, Franciscan Sister of Mill Hill, RGN, RM
Ward Sister, St Joseph's Hospice, London

Karen Slatcher, RGN
Deputy Ward Sister, St Joseph's Hospice, London

Sally Unsworth, MSc, RGN, RM, MTD, RCNT, ADM, FPC
Midwife/Nurse Manager, Bradford Hospitals

Dr Giovambattista Zeppetella, BSc, MRCGP
Medical Consultant, St Joseph's Hospice, London

Note: RSC denotes member of the Religious Sisters of Charity.

Preface

This third edition of a popular textbook has been completely revised by the joint editors, Janet Moscrop and Joy Robbins.

As in previous editions, the focus is on the person dying at home, in residential care or in hospital and the emphasis is on teamwork in caring for the individual and their relatives and friends. Experts in all aspects of care have contributed to this complete revision of the previous text and each chapter is written by a different member of the multiprofessional team.

The chapter on the terminal care of people suffering from AIDS has been enlarged and consideration is also given to care of those in the terminal stages of other non-malignant diseases. Other new material includes chapters on complementary therapy, the use of the day centre, the value of volunteers, diversional therapy and respite care.

The chapter on bereavement covers many aspects of grief and loss and there is a sensitive approach to the need for supporting staff in this specialized work. Consideration is also given to the needs of dying and grieving people from differing ethnic backgrounds with varying cultural expectations in a pluralistic society.

The third edition offers a broad overview of the support given to the dying person and the carers by medical and nursing staff, physiotherapists, pharmacists, social workers, the chaplaincy and members of the pastoral care team. Students of all these disciplines should find this book both readable and informative.

Many references for further study provide a foundation for qualified nurses seeking further experience in palliative and terminal care. The book provides a comprehensive textbook for nursing students gaining experience in this sphere and useful information for the qualified nurses supervising their studies. There are specific examples of nursing assessment based on research, on symptom control and management for inpatients and those in domiciliary care. This edition can be confidently recommended for all libraries of nursing and those of other caring professions. It should prove a stimulus for qualified nurses to deepen their skills and knowledge, which will surely enhance the care of dying patients and their families.

Sheila Collins OBE PhD BA FRCN RGN RSCN RNT
Chairperson, Board of Management, St Joseph's Hospice, London.

Acknowledgements

We wish to record with gratitude the help given by many people in the preparation of this third edition. Firstly, to Sister Helen, Matron of St Joseph's Hospice, for her encouragement and help in allowing the facilities of the Norfolk Wing Study Centre to be used. We wish to thank particularly Dhangari Halai for her patience and willingness to undertake much extra secretarial work on our behalf. We thank the editorial staff of our publishers Chapman & Hall, for their encouragement and advice. Finally, we owe a great debt of gratitude to our colleague Jennifer Clark and to all our contributors who worked so hard to produce the final manuscript, mainly as an extra task to a demanding fulltime job.

We end these acknowledgements as in previous editions: all of us owe the main inspiration for writing any part of this book to the countless dying patients and their families for whom we have been privileged to care in some way.

Note: All royalties from the sale of this book will go to St Joseph's Hospice, London.

Looking at death and dying

1

Several thousand years ago the preacher in the Book of Ecclesiastes wrote: 'There is a time to be born and a time to die', and yet though this is a certain fact, death today is a subject not discussed with ease.

Interestingly, Phillipe Aries (1974), in his extensive study on attitudes to death, identifies that, as far back as the Middle Ages, we accepted the fact that death is part of life. However, attitudes have altered over the centuries due to the changes which have arisen in society.

Today in the twentieth century there has developed a denial of death, that it is an enemy of life which has led to fear. Thus, in an attempt to understand the attitudes we have, the beliefs, the pattern of society, the way of life and all that influences it must be taken into account.

AGE AT WHICH PEOPLE DIE

Some 200 years ago it was thought well if you reached beyond childhood years as infant mortality was high. Also, most people that had survived those years died at what today we would call the prime of life. Around the middle part of the nineteenth century the life expectancy had risen to around 40+ years; in the 1930s it was 60+ years and by 1950s 70+ years. In the 1990s a man's expectancy of life is 72 years and a woman 78 years.

The rise in the standard of living is the main reason for such changes, as we have improved agricultural methods giving rise to the provision of more food and of greater variety. Likewise there is better housing, better sanitation and the population is better educated towards good health standards. Also during this century there have been tremendous advances in medicine which is another aspect of why the mortality rate has been reduced. Families, too, are smaller and much investment is made in the children as they, along with their parents, expect to have a long life. It is also a fact that much time and energy is devoted to research and therapeutic measures with the aim of reducing disease and extending life. All this has caused death to seem remote rather than the reality that it **is** a fact of life.

For some years following the Second World War we had economic recovery which in the western hemisphere was also linked to a revolution in technology. This has led people from all levels of society to avail themselves of a wide range of consumer goods which several decades ago would have been unattainable for many.

Poverty still exists in today's society, yet compared with the years between the two World Wars, there is evidence that even here there has been a measure of improvement. More people in Britain today own their own homes, most of which have a bath or shower, over half have central heating and a high percentage have more than one car per family. The age of consumerism has led to an increased pressure for people to improve on their standard of living. It is hard for us in the affluent West to comprehend the extent of deprivation and starvation leading to death that still exists in many areas of the world, even though it is constantly portrayed on television and through the media.

CAUSES AND LOCATION OF DEATH

Despite advances in medical care the main cause of death in the Western world is cardiovascular diseases, followed closely by malignant diseases and also accidents. This latter category is at its peak in the 15–44 age group and is no doubt attributable to the increase in road traffic accidents, accidents at work and also in the homicide and self-destruction rate.

This century has witnessed some horrific events, such as two World Wars, the horrors of the Nazi gas chambers, the explosion of the atom bomb at Hiroshima and the increase in international terrorism. Yet what a strange society we now live in as, in the main, we have rejected the death penalty for serious crime. On the other hand, we are constantly reminded that 'in the midst of life we are in death' as we learn of the many natural disasters which seem to occur almost daily, such as the extensive flooding in Bangladesh and massive earthquakes in Central Asia and other areas of the world.

There has been a considerable shift during this century for more people to die in an institution (currently about 70%) despite the fact that most would prefer to die in their own homes. This in turn further isolates the dying person from everyday life. Also it mean that many more reach adult life without having witnessed a natural death.

Although no age throughout history has been spared violence and violent deaths, it seems to be increasingly prevalent in our society today as there is always an area of the world where violence is present, be it wars, riots or drunken drivers. Since communications are now easier and faster worldwide, people become more readily aware of such events.

FACING FACTS OF DEATH AND DYING

In society today we appear to have developed two totally different ways of facing the issues of dying and death. It is certainly possible to read graphic newspaper accounts of sudden deaths, or long obituaries of well-known personalities who have died and yet not have negative attitudes towards death. Likewise television and radio are able to portray some of the horrifying aspects of death and yet also present well-documented programmes on bereavement and issues related to death and dying in a natural way. Generally these are well received and cover sensitively many issues from stillbirth to people who are facing their own deaths. Yet still for many of us, death is seen as an intrusion into our lives.

Modern society has led us to fear our own death and to the denial of death. This is even true of professionals who are involved with death in their everyday work, e.g. funeral directors, counsellors, etc., as portrayed by Sarah Boston (1987) who interviewed such people for the television series 'Merely Mortal'. She found that if the discussion moved towards their own deaths, there was an attempt to quickly change the subject.

However, when the subject of death arises in conversation, the majority of us have difficulty in freely expressing ourselves. Wass (1979), in *Dying: Facing the Facts* describes how we use a different vocabulary, such as the person has 'passed away', 'passed on', etc. in place of 'died'. Death in British culture remains a private issue whereas other societies have developed language enabling them to talk about it.

Sarah Boston (1987) states: 'We have not in the twentieth century been able to avoid the subject completely, but what we have done is to develop a new and evasive language'.

ATTITUDES OF THE NURSE AND OTHER CARERS

As it is a known fact that attitudes are related to behaviour, those who are involved with the care of the dying, whether nurses or other carers, need to be mindful of their own thoughts and feelings about health as these can readily affect how they care. Surely, too, our attitudes are also influenced by society's attitude to death. However, there is also the danger that our own thoughts and fears about death can be suppressed which in turn can create a barrier as we carry out our professional duties, making us more remote in our relationship with those who are dying. One way of dealing with this issue is to acknowledge our own feelings of anxiety and helplessness in meeting with other colleagues to talk things through, accepting that this is the way to grow rather than it being a symbol of weakness.

It is generally not long before those who enter a caring proftession come face to face with death. Those in the medical profession whose education has been largely centred around the knowledge of treatment or cure can, when faced with the fact that there is no cure, feel failure and helplessness especially when facing anguished relatives.

Perhaps, though, it is the nurse who is most likely to have intimate contact with death fairly soon after commencing clinical experience and also coping with distraught relatives as they face the loss of a loved one. Furthermore, the apprehension is increased as there is the need to see the face of a dead person for the first time. Generally, though, this experience is met with relief as in most instances the sight is peaceful rather than frightening. However, in major disasters and accidents, the sight and handling of mutilated bodies will be unpleasant and emotionally difficult to handle.

However, for most of us it is in the area of communication with dying patients, their relatives and friends where the greatest difficulties arise as we try to acquire attitudes which will be of help. Here it is helpful to remember that actions speak louder than words and if physical care is carried out gently and quietly yet in an effective manner, it will demonstrate a positive attitude. Likewise a simple act of courtesy to a tired and anxious relative bestowed in an unhurried manner will convey a caring attitude.

In this respect we need to remember to be available to listen with undivided attention and respond to the best of our ability. If necessary this may mean finding help from another source, such as a more experienced colleague who may be able to continue to listen or offer help in other ways. Above all, conveying warmth and a positive attitude enables the patient to feel surrounded by a natural and pleasant atmosphere yet without a sense of false optimism.

It has been noted and mentioned at a recent Royal College of Nursing Cancer Society meeting that those who possess a religious faith can gain an inner strength, which in turn helps them in the care they give to patients and families in distress. Also the carer may have a greater insight into the emotions and needs of a family who are grieving due to a bereavement they have suffered. [This need not necessarily have been the loss of a family member but for example, a broken engagement or loss of self-esteem can actually identify some of the pain that is experienced from a bereavement.] Time is needed to reflect on such experiences and to share with experienced colleagues, as this enables helpful attitudes to develop.

It is a fact for all of us that death is a mystery but for many the fear of dying is greater than the fear of death. This had led to an avoidance of these issues, with no allowance for expression of the fears and loneliness associated with dying. Slowly this is now changing and the need to acknowledge approaching death is gradually being accepted as a necessity, though sadly in some areas in the western world this is only just beginning to happen.

Education, both for student nurses and more recently for medical students, does include aspects such as communicating with the dying and the bereaved. Likewise, this need is being met in continuing education, the Open University, for example, having recently produced a package on death, dying and bereavement (Dickenson and Johnson, 1993). Thus with increasing education, observing experienced colleagues at work, making use of the literature that is now more readily available and also making an effort to overcome the tendency to avoid the dying patient due to our own feelings of pain and inadequacy, we can express a confident attitude to our dying patients.

IS THERE LIFE AFTER DEATH?

In previous centuries this question would not have been publicly raised. Archaeologists have provided irrefutable evidence from antiquity that the dead were provided with articles of everyday living to sustain them on their journey to the next life. Written and oral traditions from every part of the world reinforce this fundamental belief although the perceived nature of the afterlife varies greatly. European history, with its Christian roots as a major influence, has consistently shown a belief in the resurrection of the body and the immortality of the soul. Death is thus seen as only a gateway to eternal life.

The awesome advances in scientific knowledge and the decline in universal religious practice and belief in the twentieth century have produced a major change in formulating attitudes to the leading question – is there life after death? In dealing with such complex issues, it is only possible here to summarize the situation found in the UK. There appear to be three types of attitudes:

1. A firm belief in an afterlife among those who practise a particular religious faith with a full acceptance of all its tenets. The exact nature of this afterlife is recognized by many to be unclear.
2. An open mind on the subject, not ruling out the possibility but with no definite conviction. Some people in this group may be nominally

Christian and in facing their own death when the time comes, may seek help in sorting out their attitudes. Others remain agnostic till the end.

3. Those who are quite clear that for them death is the absolute end of human existence, except for the memories that people leave behind of themselves.

Because these different standpoints may change throughout a person's life, including the last days, there is no exactitude about proportions of people holding a certain attitude at any one time.

There is an increasing interest in connection with this matter in what is known as near death experience. Due to the improvements in medical science more people than ever before are returned from the threshold of death, though many scientists are sceptical even to the point of being dismissive. However, some now believe that these events need to be considered seriously. It is now estimated that at least 1% of the population in Britain can relate having a near death experience.

It is interesting to note that these experiences appear to have a similarity. Most people felt they were losing consciousness and that they were entering a long tunnel through which they floated towards a bright light, which seemed to exude warmth, love and friendliness. While they were floating they were able to look down on their physical body and were able to discuss later, in minute details, the resuscitation procedures which were taking place. These activities were then confirmed by those who were in attendance.

Increasing interest has led to research being undertaken into near death experiences. Dr Peter Fenwick, a neuropsychiatrist and a leading clinical authority on these events, admits that they appear to confound all that we currently know about how the brain functions. Basically there is no scientific definition of what it is like to **be** a human being even though we known anatomically the working of the nervous system.

One outstanding feature of these near death experiences is in the fact that all who recall such happenings state how their lives have been profoundly affected. They all talk of a renewed sense of life's values and its preciousness and of much less interest in material gains. Also that this experience has banished their fear of death.

All this surely underlines the moral and ethical issues which have sprung from the great religious traditions. Some researchers, such as Paul Badham from the University of Dyfed, now believe that these near death experiences do confirm that there is life after death. For many who have been through this event, it has led to an increase in their religious faith.

REFERENCES

Aries, P. (1974) *Western Attitudes to Death from the Middle Ages to the Present*, Johns Hopkins University Press, Baltimore.
Boston, S. (1987) *Merely Mortal*, Methuen, London, p. 14.
Dickenson, D. and Johnson, M. (eds) (1993) *Death, Dying and Bereavement*, Sage Publications/Open University, Milton Keynes.
Ecclesiastes, Ch 3, Vs 2.
Wass, H. (1979) *Dying: Facing the Facts*, Hemisphere Publishing Corporation, London.

FURTHER READING

Doyle, D., Hanks, G.W.C. and MacDonald, N. (1993) *Oxford Textbook of Palliative Medicine*, Oxford Medical Publications, Oxford.
Office of Health Economics (1991) *Dying with dignity*, OHE, London.

2 The importance of communications with the patient, family and professional carers

> Most of what we do is dependent on our ability to send, receive and interpret signals between each other.
>
> (John Casson, 1968)

Probably the first message received by a small baby as he is expelled from his mother's body is that sent by the midwife or doctor. Hopefully the person assisting him into the world will handle him firmly but with gentleness and care as he is cleaned up, provoked to cry and wrapped up in a warm towel or blanket. It would be good to think the message transmitted to the baby is "You are safe in my hands and I am concerned for your welfare". The baby is then, normally, given to his mother who will hold him close to her, cuddle and kiss him, murmur sweet things to him, sending the message 'I love you, I want you, I need you'.

As people grow, learn to speak and acquire many skills, the ways used to send messages become more varied and complex. However, the need to send clear messages and to understand with clarity those received remains as important throughout one's life as it did in the first few hours following birth.

The baby has to learn to signal that he is hungry, uncomfortable, in pain, frightened. These signals need to elicit a prompt and correct response.

Many messages are conveyed non-verbally – body posture, facial expressions, gesticulations, touch, soft soothing sounds. It could be claimed more non-verbal messages are transmitted than those employing words. Words, and particularly choice of words, are of course important too, indeed a necessity in certain situations. But the way in which these words are uttered, the gesticulations and facial expressions which accompany them are often more significant than the words themselves.

In this chapter three different types of communications are to be examined:

1. nurse with patient;
2. nurse with relatives and other carers;
3. communication with professional carers and their attitudes to one another.

NURSE COMMUNICATING WITH PATIENT

On admission to hospital or hospice many terminally ill people will be apprehensive, anxious about pain, suffering, unpleasant procedures, loss of identity, status, dignity, separation from family and loved ones. Some are so ill they will scarcely be aware of their surroundings. They will be glad to receive a kind welcome, be transferred to a bed, their symptoms relieved if appropriate and allowed to lie quietly undisturbed, without having to make an effort of any kind. It is difficult to imagine how a very ill person feels unless or until this has been experienced. One can only surmise.

For those who are conscious, perhaps well enough to walk in and at least able to take in their surroundings, it is somewhat different. They will intimate their anxiety in a number of ways: anxious expression, eyes full of apprehension, nervous voice, tense muscles, clutching belongings or blankets tightly.

It is imperative the nurse receiving the patient allays fears, promotes confidence and makes the person feel welcomed. To receive a patient as one would a guest is a good way to start. In normal everyday situations, social or business, a warm greeting does much to reassure people and put them at ease. A friendly tone of voice, appropriate choice of words, a smile expressing interest and a welcoming gesture usually create a good first impression.

Too often, in an endeavour to be caring, especially with very ill people, nurses can sound patronizing and rather as if talking to a child. No matter how ill, the patient is still a person, an adult who until recently made his own decisions. He will appreciate being spoken to in the way normal between two adults.

It is important to give the patient a feeling of being in control. Many terminally ill people have sustained several major losses. Being ill has completely taken over their lives. They have lost freedom of choice in various areas of life on account of altered bodily functions and abilities, e.g reduced mobility. Social activities, pastimes, hobbies, work associations have been given up. With increasing weakness and disability it is vital the patient feels he is still considered to be a person, able to choose for himself.

While discussing the patient's own particular situation to identify main difficulties and preferences it is advisable to conduct this in a low voice which excludes unwilling eavesdroppers. How many patients must find distasteful the questions, asked in a clear penetrating voice, relating to bodily functions. Most patients are not deaf and when deafness is a problem extra care is required to ensure privacy.

When explaining routines to the patient it is essential to use words which will be readily understood.

Attitudes towards people can be based on erroneous assumptions which dictate the behaviour adopted by one person towards another, e.g. those belonging to a high or low social class, clerical/manual, professional status, etc. It is dangerous to assume things and more so, to act accordingly, especially when trying to work out how people would prefer to be treated.

Altered body image may have resulted in gross disfigurement. The nurse must conceal shock, disgust or revulsion if someone's appearance is grotesque or odd. This also applies to certain habits practised by the patient or even style of dress, hair, etc.

However, if these are too irregular or it is though they may offend other patients and/or their relatives then the issue must be tackled with tact and diplomacy. The patient must be made to realize his behaviour or appearance is socially unacceptable.

In dealings with patients and relatives the cardinal rule should at all times be impartiality. Most carers do have a natural tendency towards particular people rather than others but this should not be in evidence. To accept each patient for who he is is of utmost importance. So often terminally ill people admit to feeling they have been abandoned – because no further treatment can avail a cure. In the hospital or hospice, caring staff can reverse this situation and help people to feel wanted and loved, accepted. While cure may not be possible much healing can occur, healing of emotional, social and spiritual pains and scars. As Mr Oddling Smee, a surgeon, has said, 'There is always something we can do for our patients – even up until the moment after death' (Working with the Terminally Ill, video, Tavistock Publications).

When attending to the physical needs of patients, e.g. hygiene or nutritional, great sensitivity to the feelings of the patient is required. What is felt by the patient may seldom be expressed. Not many people would voluntarily sit on a commode screened off by flimsy curtains or permit another person to wash intimate parts of the body, attend to teeth, dentures or feed them. Yet this is just what the seriously ill person has to contend with and accept – dependence upon other people because he is too weak to perform these tasks for himself. It is a great privilege to be allowed to touch and care for someone else's body. Nurses are in the unique position of being permitted to do so. Everything the nurse says and does while performing these services communicates care, esteem, love, empathy and conversely a lack of these qualities. In preserving the integrity and dignity of the patient the nurse, in essence, supplies the patient's deepest needs and accomplishes the ideal in nursing.

Listening and Responding to the Patient

At all times the nurse should try to give the patient the impression she has time to stay beside him, listen to what he has to say and answer his questions. Only then will the patient have an opportunity to unburden himself. Listening is one of the most necessary of all skills for the nurse to develop. If insufficient time is available at that moment the nurse should say so and promise to come back later. This commitment must then be honoured. However, if the patient's need is immediate the nurse must decide if later will be too late and act accordingly.

> Listening is an attitude towards other people and what they are attempting to express. It begins with attention, both the outward manifestation and the inward alertness . . . tries to hear everything that is said, not just what he expects or wants to hear.
>
> (Campbell, 1984)

Much is written today about the failure of doctors and nurses to communicate adequately with dying people and the reasons for this. It is helpful to have thought through one's own attitudes to dying and to be comfortable with these thoughts. Most people, including doctors and nurses, have experienced losses in some form or other – 'lost' relationships, failure in examinations or career expectations/aspirations, loss, through death even, of a close friend, relative or pet. So it is possible to use these experiences and the emotions accompanying them to explore with the patient the nature and meaning of his very personal losses. The stages of grief are similar whatever the cause.

In law a practitioner must not lie to the patient. Also, information about the patient's condition should not be disclosed to relatives or others without the patient's permission. The relationship between a patient and the practitioner is confidential and while the latter may withhold information in the patient's best interests this information should not then be divulged to other parties.

It is always possible to be truthful without overwhelming the patient with the whole unpalatable truth. The enquiring patient needs to be given correct information regarding his condition and life expectancy. The nurse can try to ascertain what the patient already knows by asking simple questions such as 'What do you know about your illness?' or 'What have you been given to understand about your illness?'. Patients who are not improving but on the contrary are deteriorating, perhaps developing new symptoms, generally suspect all is not well and arrive at the truth themselves.

As Robin Downie, Professor of Moral Philosophy, Glasgow, said in a lecture, 'When the surveyor is called in we expect him to reveal the presence of dry rot, if it is present, and will be angry should he fail to do so'. (Lisa Sainsbury Foundation Symposium, 'Caring for Dying People', Queen Elizabeth Conference Centre, 21 September 1989).

There is now plenty of evidence to indicate it is beneficial to discuss with the patient the realistic outcomes of his illness. Patients are relieved to have an opportunity to bring their fears out into the open where there is mutual trust and understanding. Patients often express highly improbable fears such as 'I'm afraid I'll bleed to death', 'I'm afraid I'll suffocate to death', 'I'm afraid I'll never see my home and garden again'. One patient about to be married had to wait for a larger wedding ring to be made for him. He asked, 'Do you think I'll pop off before it's ready?' A woman prior to going home for a weekend break asked, 'Will it be all right for me to have intercourse with my husband?'. To all of these a sensitive nurse can respond with reassurance that worst fears will almost certainly not be realized.

Some patients who are known to have a strong religious faith can be encouraged to make that faith work. One woman, a devout Roman Catholic, experienced severe paroxysms of fear but was unable to say exactly what occasioned these. The nurse asked if the priest visited and was told the patient celebrated mass regularly. The nurse then reminded the patient of the promise made by Christ to his followers: 'I will never leave you nor forsake you' and the many occasions when he urged people to 'Fear not, be not afraid'. The patient thought about these for some minutes, gradually regained her composure and said she was greatly comforted.

In the hospice especially, patients are much relieved when they see other people, more ill, receiving care and attention right up until after death has occurred. In most cases the end of life is peaceful, without drama. This promotes confidence. People are given the very real hope that their death too, when it comes, will be calm, without suffering.

NURSE COMMUNICATING WITH RELATIVES AND OTHER CARERS

The relatives and other close friends are often as anxious as the patient when the latter is admitted. Many people are afraid in particular of the word 'hospice' and believe still it is the last port of call, the place to which people go when death approaches. This, of course, is one of the biggest misunderstandings. However it is not possible, should a hospice be involved, immediately to convince people otherwise. Often relatives are reluctant to relinguish their part in caring for the sick person who may have been, until recent events, more than adequately looked after at home. Thus relatives sometimes have a complex array of emotions including guilt at abandoning the patient, bitterness, anger and fear and therefore careful handling is required. However, even in this situation relatives can be encouraged to be involved with the care of the patient, if they desire. They need truthful information about the patient's condition and prognosis. There is no easy way to break bad news. Bad news is painful and alters a person's perception of the future. The greater the gap between reality and a person's expectations of the future the more painful is the bad news (R. Buckman, Why Won't They Talk to Me?, video, Norwich Eaton Ltd, Linkward Productions). No matter how bad the news it should be accompanied by hope. Hope can mean different things to different people and varies with the situation. According to Robert Twycross, hope is an expectation greater than zero of achieving a goal (International Cancer Conference, London, 3rd September 1988).

While some people may be devastated by the prospect of death in the near future others may be more fearful of prolongation of life with increasing disability and perhaps altered mental state. So on the one hand some relatives need help in coming to terms with death sooner than expected while on the other hand people need to be reassured that the end will not be too long in coming. Predictions of life expectancy are more often than not inaccurate. Nursing and medical staff alike would be wise to avoid making any such prognosis.

On admission of the patient the relatives should be made to feel welcome, offered hospitality and given the opportunity to assist the patient into bed or chair and to unpack his belongings. They require guidance about visiting, meal and rest times. They need reassurances they were welcome to help in the patient's care if this is desired. Some relatives and patients appreciate this, others seem happier if nursing staff take over.

In a hospice the atmosphere generally is more relaxing and homelike than a hospital because there is no 'to and fro' between busy departments.

Relatives must be given privacy when talking with the patient, which may necessitate screening the bed.

Usually, the proposed care and treatment of the patient is discussed with the patient himself and his closest relative or carer. In this way options available can be put forward and patients and relative have a chance to exercise choice.

Relatives need to be told they can telephone or enquire at any time and reassured they will be contacted should the patient's condition deteriorate. Many hospitals and hospices now have overnight facilities, guest rooms in or near the clinical areas. However, when death is imminent the closest relative or friend often does not want to remove himself from the bedside. A comfortable chair should be provided. In cases where, at the end, death seems to be delayed, the relative may need to be encouraged to take a short break. It sometimes happens that at this very moment, when the relative is absent, the patient dies. This can be extremely upsetting for the relative who may need much support and comfort.

Although many relatives have prepared themselves for the event it can still be a great shock for some when death actually occurs. It may have taken days, weeks, months and in some instances, years before a person, pronounced terminally ill, finally dies. Patients are admitted who look as if they may not survive more than a day or two at most. With modern palliative care symptoms abate and people take on a renewed lease of life. When this happens it can be a mixed blessing. Relatives and patients are given additional time together. Patients may attend day centres, learn new creative hobbies and skills, make new friends. People can be lulled into thinking they are 'better', if not cured. Indeed, they are 'better' but the disease process moves inexorably on towards the inevitable which can be later rather than sooner. So relatives have 'to readjust to death all over again', as one relative expressed it.

Sometimes, too, patients die suddenly and occasionally from something other than the terminal disease. In these situations the nurse, more than ever, needs to respond sensitively to the relative, communicating feelings by means of gestures and touch rather than words. Words often seem totally inadequate at such a time but it is often soothing to the relative if the nurse can make some kind, complimentary remark about the patient, e.g. 'Your husband was such a thoughtful man, friendly and helpful to other patients. We all liked him'. Or simply to say, 'I am so sorry/sad your wife has died'.

Relatives, too, need the time to talk about their worries. In today's society divorce and separation are common. It is equally common for a couple who are not married to live together. In the circle of relatives and friends surrounding the patient there can be a variety of relationships. Within these there can be tension leading to bitterness, resentment and jealousy. Financial problems may exist. When relationships are strained and unhappy, whatever the cause, relatives or friends may be glad when the patient dies and this can give rise to guilt feelings; guilt because there is neither regret nor sadness, only immense relief.

Tension and anxiety can have repercussions on the patient, whose symptoms may be aggravated. It is not possible for caring staff to resolve or ease all family problems but by adopting an unhurried approach and giving time to listen, recognizing and acknowledging the intense feelings expressed, much can be done to defuse volatile situations.

Good care of the patient conveys comforting messages to relatives who can see him receiving attention, i.e. being washed, hair combed, teeth/dentures and mouth cleaned, position in bed changed, fresh linen on the bed, clean night clothes, right up until after death.

When Death Occurs and Immediately Thereafter

While screening off a bed prior to or immediately following death is frowned upon by some, it nevertheless affords privacy for relatives who may not want to say their farewells under the public gaze.

Sometime a relative likes a nurse to stay beside the bed until the patient has died. As mentioned earlier it is not necessary to say many words at such a time. It suffices to have the presence of another person, especially, perhaps, a professional to whom one can look for support.

It is the usual custom for relatives to return home until the following day when the death certificate and other formalities are completed.

A small quiet room should be at the disposal of relatives for the purpose of giving information with regard to registering the death, obtaining the services of a funeral director and to receive the personal effects of the deceased. A nurse closest to the patient and/or family should be available to perform this service, perhaps the named nurse. Again, this admits a personal element to what might otherwise be a routine formality.

It is deplorable that, in certain hospitals, relatives are obliged to go to a central office. This is a highly impersonal way of managing this event. Relatives want contact with people who actually provided care for the patient. They need to talk to those who last attended the patient. They need to hear about the circumstances in which the patient died, how he died, the last words, if any, that were uttered, if the relatives themselves were not present at the time of death.

Relatives/friends should be invited to see the deceased if they have not done so. Indeed, they should be encouraged to do so. For most people it is something they want to do. They should be permitted as much time as required.

The patient's body will have been washed and dressed in clean clothes and requests for special attire should be complied with. Perhaps more thought should be given to offering relatives the opportunity of helping in these last aspects of care.

All of the above may appear simple but to grieving people aware that their needs are being considered, they are immensely important.

Early Bereavement

Following the death of a loved one most people, though sad and lonely, gradually resume a normal life routine into which new friendships, social and recreational interests are introduced. For these people it is sufficient to assure them that ward staff can always be contacted should they find things difficult. But for others the grieving process is more drawn out. Loneliness is unbearable. Conflicting emotions sweep through them. The feeling they will never adjust to the change is predominant. Many hospitals and hospices offer a support service to bereaved relatives and friends which can be of inestimable value. Regular group meetings are arranged under the supervision of an experienced counsellor to which relatives are invited. They can then share with others their feelings and experience.

While it may not be advisable as a general rule for staff to attend funerals or make bereavement visits, it may sometimes be perfectly in order. Not all relatives/carers would wish for, or expect it, but many patients are cared for at home with a community sister or MacMillan nurse visiting frequently. Carers come to regard these professionals as friends. When close bonds have been formed it can be an additional upset if all contact with the nurse ceases on the demise of the patient. Memories of the funeral well attended, familiar faces present, letters received containing kind words about the deceased can sustain and strengthen relatives for some considerable time.

So much of a person's skill in communicating depends on a natural, spontaneous, warm response to another's needs in varied circumstances. The attitudes of professional carers will make a lasting impression on the minds of family members and friends.

COMMUNICATION WITH PROFESSIONAL CARERS AND THEIR ATTITUDES TO ONE ANOTHER

Communication with patients, family and friends will only be effective if the professionals communicate effectively with each other.

Communicating is a means by which one person respects another.

> . . . it links human beings at both verbal and non-verbal levels of interaction. Failure to communicate or refusal turns the other person into a thing – an inanimate object which can be manipulated in ways that suit us.

So says Campbell (1984) in his book *Moral Dilemmas in Medicine*.

In nursing, especially today, much emphasis is placed on team nursing. What is a team? A group with a common goal. 'Two or more persons working together – willingness to act as a member of a group rather than an individual' (*Concise Oxford Dictionary*).

However, a team may not necessarily imply teamwork! In any team the various members employ different skills to achieve a common purpose. Every member is essential for efficient team functioning. A team member communicates his intentions to others. Where there is mutual trust and confidence the less skilled or less experienced will more readily seek guidance and help from senior staff.

These attitudes should extend to include all members of the interdisciplinary team, e.g. cleaning, catering, maintenance, administrative, clerical, secretarial, chaplaincy, physiotherapy, counsellors, social workers and medical and nursing staff. When a team really pulls together people help each other, ungrudgingly. Petty grumbling should be almost nonexistent. People will be aware of the needs and commitments of others.

For example, a nurse is required to sit down and listen to a patient who has urgent matters to discuss. The nurse should not be called upon to do something which can be accomplished equally well by someone else. Very often a patient will relate better to someone who is on the same social level. A ward sister revealed that the cleaner is often better able to cope with certain patients than nursing staff.

Staff communications and attitudes towards colleagues are not one sided. More senior members of the team, like everyone else, need encouragement, need to feel useful and appreciate support from others. These people too have bad days, difficult situations with which to contend which can affect their behaviour towards their peers or subordinates.

Professionals are continually urged to adopt a holistic approach to their patients. One must remember too that staff are whole people. They have interests, abilities, facets which all add up to the complete person and this is reflected in everything he does and in his relationships.

Professionals, too, must listen to each other. They need to have time for each other. Too often staff are so concerned about the needs of patients and families they think nothing of breaking off or interrupting a conversation with a fellow worker. Unless it is an emergency or urgent situation there is no reason why common courtesies cannot be accorded to colleagues. It all hinges yet again on respecting persons, whoever these may be.

THE SELF-IMAGE

This section cannot be complete without making mention of the self-image.

The self-image is how a person perceives himself to be or how he would like to be. If the discrepancy between perception and reality is too great the self-image is false and this adversely affects the way in which a person communicates with others. Afraid that people may see him as he really is, the person attempts to hide his deficiencies, as they appear to him. He acts a part, shields behind a façade and therefore never shows himself as he really is. So, to avoid this people must come to terms with who and what they are. They have to appraise themselves, acknowledge their good and bad points. This applies to everything – physical appearance, mannerisms, dialect, background (social and educational), personal attributes and characteristics.

The person who can be content with himself as he is, and with his possessions, will be more able to communicate well with others because he has nothing to conceal.

This chapter ends with the personal account of one lady's sentiments. Although she is not terminally ill it provides a salutary lesson to all involved in health care.

> While I was in hospital for insertion of radium wires I had a heavy period. I was embarrassed when a young male student nurse introduced himself as my nurse for the night. There was no way I was going to allow him to remove my commode pan (she was of course in isolation) and so I went all night without going to the toilet. I waited until morning but was dismayed to find, when finally I did go, he was still on duty. There was nothing really wrong with him. It was me, my attitude. It was routine for him.

The same lady went on to say:

> There is far too much talk about cancer today and the reactions and feelings one is supposed to have. It is assumed when you are told you have cancer you will be shocked, devastated and that you will experience certain feelings. In my case it was not a shock. After all, one goes to the doctor who tells you a second opinion is needed. You see a consultant, have a mammogram, a needle is stuck in your breast, you are told you need a biopsy. Alarm bells have been ringing for some time so it is no surprise when finally you are told.
>
> I did not have the negative thoughts I was expected to have. The counsellor puts negative thoughts into your head and then does nothing about it. I was not horrified by the result of my surgery. I had part of my breast removed. It is not pretty but I still have a breast and I don't like or wear the false part. I only wish they'd taken some off the other breast.
>
> Magazines and papers print these horror stories because they need to sell.

All the doctors and nurses were level and kept me well informed throughout of all that was going on and the options available were presented for me to make my choice. But I did not want to know all the ins and outs and I did not want to discuss it with other patients or hear from them what they had or did. I just wanted to get on with my life.

'Communicate – to transmit information, thought or feeling so that it is satisfactorily received or understood' (Wilkinson, 1991). This must be high on the list of priorities of all health care staff, especially those caring for dying patients and their families.

REFERENCES

Campbell, A. (1984) *Moral Dilemmas in Medicine*, 3rd edn, Churchill Livingstone, Edinburgh.

Casson, J. (1968) *Using Words*, Duckworth, London.

Wilkinson, J. (1991) The ethics of communication in palliative care. *Palliative Medicine*, **5**, 130–7.

FURTHER READING

Buckman, R. (1988) *I Don't Know What to Say*, Papermac, London.

Buckman, R. (1992) *How to Break Bad News*, Papermac, London.

Hinton, J. (1991) *Dying*, Penguin, Harmondsworth.

Kübler-Ross, E. (1970) *On Death and Dying*, Tavistock, London.

Lamerton, R. (1973) *Care of the Dying*, Penguin, Harmondsworth.

Lichter, I. (1987) *Communication in Cancer Care*, Churchill Livingstone, Edinburgh.

3 Nursing assessment

The nursing assessment in palliative care, whether performed at home or in a hospice setting, is of paramount importance because we are aiming to provide a quality of life that is acceptable to the patient.

Much has been written and researched over recent years on the nursing assessment issue and this must be greatly welcomed, as it is a real attempt to equip nurses with the tools and skills to provide the optimal standard of care for all patients, but most particularly for the terminally ill. Developing a nursing assessment tool for dying patients is a complicated task, because we are preparing patients not for life and health but for a peaceful death with dignity. We may care for patients who we can properly assess and for whom we can implement a structured care plan, but our attempts to do so may be thwarted if the prognosis is less than 48 hours and a proportionately high number of problems exist. It is then vital to deal with those that greatly affect the patient's comfort and give what support is necessary for the family. The point in question here is that the nursing assessment process must allow flexibility for all situations.

It follows then that a philosophy of care is central to any nursing assessment. Johns (1989) suggests that a philosophy for practice arises as a result of an exploration and agreement of minds about what nursing is in relation to the realities of shared practice. Johns also goes on to discuss that where staff share a belief about nursing within their workplace the care is more likely to be consistent and of real benefit to the patients.

So the philosophy ideally should reflect the common values of the nursing team; this in reality is difficult to achieve because of the diversity of human thinking and feeling, levels of expertise and skill mix. Also in a multidisciplinary approach, which is the essence of palliative care, other disciplines may create a challenge to the nursing philosophy. It is still widely felt that doctors control the patient's treatment. Research by Field (1984) shows that doctors can and do impose restrictions on the care offered by nurses. In palliative care, however, where medicine fails to provide a cure, the combined nursing and medical expertise can provide a quality of life that is of utmost importance.

The model of nursing used in palliative care should reflect the philosophy for practice, even if that means creating one's own model. An excellent example was the Burford experiment (Johns, 1991) where a model was devised based on questions. It seemed to allow for exploration instead of questioning, ensuring that all aspects of care were covered but it also allowed for the nurse to care for the patient as an individual and also remain within the confines of the model most widely used in assessing and caring for patients. In a research project, McCaugherty (1992) has showed how this model has held up to the scrutiny of research in its ability to help learners relate theory to practice. Other models may provide an equally accurate nursing assessment, but the Activities of Living model (Roper, Logan and Tierney, 1983) has a very strong relevance in palliative care and it is on this model that the description of the care will be based in this nursing assessment chapter.

ASSESSMENT OF THE DYING PATIENT

First meeting with the patient

First impressions are crucial in any situation where two people are hoping to build up a relationship. The nurse works with the patient on a basis of concern and understanding. Allowing the patient to exercise control in decision making where possible can only enhance the relationship between nurse and patient. This should include the family and friends and whatever else forms the patient's social and cultural existence. The nurse's aim is to gather essential information by observation, examination and conversation with the patient and family. The dying patient, through his vulnerability, will be looking for certain characteristics in the nurse. A study (Hull, 1991) revealed these to be effective communication skills, caring, non-judgemental attitude and being a competent practitioner who is accessible 24 hours a day.

If these skills and qualities are not apparent to the patient, either subconsciously or otherwise, then the assessment and the development of the nurse–patient relationship may be hindered.

The nurse's manner of approach

A research study (Ashworth, 1980) refers to the positive effect on human interaction of physical proximity, eye contact, a friendly tone of voice and conversation about personal topics. The nurse establishing contact with the dying patient can make use of these findings as follows.

1. By sitting close to the patient, by the bed or chair where it is easy to talk face to face. A smile and friendly greeting should be appropriate.
2. By attention to the tone of voice and conversation. The patient may not be able to hear well, whether through age or weakness, so that a clear measured mode of speech helps. Courtesy shown by addressing the patient by his or her correct title and warmth of tone imply concern and interest.
3. Touch is a powerful source of social bonding and the nurse should take the patient's hand in the initial greeting. Where it seems helpful, as with a patient who is obviously distressed and anxious, the nurse should not hesitate to hold the patient's hand gently for a time.

These initial steps to establish contact are very important to the dying patient in showing that care will include the unhurried offering of time by his or her professional carers, especially in being prepared to listen.

Obtaining information

Having established contact and expended effort in gaining the patient's confidence, the nurse using the model for practice can gain the information she needs to provide the appropriate care. Observation and examination are also important parts of the initial assessment. It is possible that the patient may be able to answer only a few questions due to confusion, weakness, pain or any of the other distressing symptoms that may be seen and it is here that the family may provide necessary information. This also gives the family time to express their own emotional anxieties. If they have the opportunity to unburden themselves then the nurse–family bond of trust has begun to develop.

One factor that is of particular importance for all those caring for the dying patient is the extent of insight that the patient appears to have into the nature and prognosis of his or her illness. Today, many patients are well informed as to their diagnosis and prognosis and may volunteer this information readily. Others, however, may have been told but within the process of grieving they may still be denying what is happening. Professionals within the palliative care field should have a clear understanding of the bereavement process as clearly defined by Parkes (1982). Lack of knowledge in this may lead to a misinterpretation of an angry response from a patient.

Assessing whether patients understand that they are dying is often difficult and needs time for a relationship to be established between patients and carers. On the other hand some patients will make their thoughts clear at the onset, in direct statements about their approaching demise or in a firm optimism about an eventual cure. This information should be recorded, whether it has been obtained by the nurse or another colleague,

Table 3.1 Activities of living

Maintaining a safe environment
Communicating
Breathing
Eating and drinking
Eliminating
Personal cleansing and dressing
Controlling body temperature
Mobilizing
Working and playing
Expressing sexuality
Sleeping
Dying

so that all the team are aware of the extent of the patient's insight into his or her condition.

The practical details required during the initial assessment are aptly covered in the Roper *et al.* Activities of Daily Living model (Table 3.1). This information may be obtained over a period of time, which will involve getting to know the patient. Any worries expressed regarding finance or family welfare may be brought to the attention of the social workers. Spiritual and religious beliefs may or may not be of importance to the patient, but respecting the individual's wishes in this area is very important.

In a multicultural society it is important to have the aid of an interpreter, as the anxieties of the patient will increase, as will feelings of isolation, if every effort is not made to communicate properly.

Observation of the patient

The nurse can learn much by observing the patient during the initial contact, as the following examples will demonstrate:

1. **Facial expression.** This may reflect pain, anxiety, apathy, hostility, depression, which will give a clue to underlying problems both physical and psychological. On the other hand, the patient may appear serene and smiling. People may mask their feelings so that superficial observation of the face does not reveal the true state of affairs. It is thus helpful to try to see patient 'off guard' before or after actually meeting them face to face.
2. **Position in bed/chair.** Many dying patients prefer to be out of bed for

part of the day and even walking about until weakness overwhelms the power of mobility. Posture can again reveal emotional problems such as depression or anxiety and certainly pain. The patient may be sitting or lying in an unnatural position with contorted limbs. If walking about, the degree of agility can be noted. The depressed patient may be hunched up with bent head or hidden under the bedclothes. Anxiety or confusion is often accompanied by restlessness and twisting of the hands.

3. **Odour.** On approaching the patient, the nurse may be aware of an odour that gives a clue to a particular problem. The smell of faeces or urine alerts one to a situation of incontinence or a badly controlled stoma. The patient may not actually be vomiting at the time, but contamination of personal clothing by vomit on a previous occasion may not have been dealt with adequately and leaves a typical lingering odour. The presence of a fungating wound is not uncommon, especially in advanced breast cancer, and will certainly have an unpleasant odour that may be apparent even when the wound is not exposed.
4. **Sounds.** Respiratory symptoms are common in the dying patient so that the nurse may hear the patient coughing, breathing noisily or, if death is near and secretions that the patient cannot expel are filling the trachea, the so-called 'death rattle'. In listening to the patient, the nurse may notice a speech impediment, such as slurring, or hoarseness of voice.
5. **Level of consciousness.** When first meeting a dying patient, a wide range of mental states will be observed. Some patients remain alert and conscious right up to the moments before death occurs. This can be the case in the terminal stage of a chronic illness as well as in sudden and unexpected death.

   In a chronic illness, most patients lapse into coma during the last few hours, if not earlier. A semiconscious state is common during the last 48 hours, especially during the terminal stage of a malignant disease. The nurse may realize that the patient is confused to some degree and unable to give reliable verbal information.

Physical examination of the patient

This should be done gently and unobtrusively and starts with the first attempt to make the patient comfortable in bed or chair and later when dealing with skin, toilet and other aspects of physical care. Specific observations will include:

- colour, texture and integrity of skin and mucous membranes;
- presence of swellings in any part of the body;

- oedema or muscle wasting;
- abnormal position of limbs;
- unusual movements such as shaking or trembling;
- incontinence of urine or faeces;
- level of consciousness and orientation.

The nurse will, of course, gain further information from the doctor's findings such as the result of rectal or vaginal examination, abdominal palpation and the quality of cardiac and respiratory function. The nurse should also be aware of the signs of impending death as his or her first contact with the patient may be at a late stage in the terminal illness (Chapter 6).

ASSESSMENT OF THE FAMILY

All those caring for dying patients must consider them within the context of a family unit, however small. When patients appear to have no living family or friends, their professional carers must become their 'family' to some extent.

Details of the initial care of the family when patients are at home are given in Chapter 16. The following guidelines are offered for nurses who are dealing with the family when patients are admitted for residential care. A methodological history should be taken to obtain the fullest information possible, including the family's perception of the patient's problems and the part that they have so far played in looking after him or her. As with patients, nurses should be alert in observing signs of anxiety, fatigue and exhaustion, even actual ill health in family members. The interview may take place while the doctor is elsewhere assessing the patient. A warm, sympathetic approach on the nurse's part and provision of a cup of tea is a good beginning to forging a relationship. Relatives often express guilt that they have allowed the patient to be removed from home and positive reassurance that they can continue to help in other ways is important.

After the doctor has seen the patient he or she will talk with the relatives together with the nurse and a simple, clear explanation of the patient's condition should be given together with the likely prognosis. The relatives should have the opportunity to ask questions and should be told that they are welcome to visit at any time or to telephone. They should be assured that they may stay the night if they wish. A telephone number where the next-of-kin can be reached should be obtained. Enquiries regarding the religious faith of the patient should be made and any special requests carefully noted. Information about the religious practices and beliefs of the main world religions will be found in Chapters 6 and

13. If the patient has been admitted at an already late stage of illness, the relatives should be informed of the likely changes during the next days or hours and asked if they wish to be present at the time of death. Some relatives do not wish to be at the bedside then and their wishes must be respected.

This chapter has set out the first stages of the process of nursing dying patients and their families, i.e. assessment. Subsequent chapters will deal with establishing nursing goals, giving appropriate care and evaluating its effectiveness, while further chapters have been written by professional colleagues who are experts in other aspects of care, such as medicine and social work. There will be some overlap between all the writers, which will serve to reinforce important points and also to reflect the fact that, to be successful, the care of dying patients and their families is a team effort that people share for a common goal, namely, death in peace, comfort and dignity.

REFERENCES

Ashworth, P. (1980) *Care to Communicate*, Royal College of Nursing, London.

Field, D. (1984) We didn't want him to die on his own – nurses' accounts of nursing dying patients. *Journal of Advanced Nursing*, **9**(1), 59–70.

Hull, M. (1991) Hospice nurses (Caring support for caregiving families). *Journal of Cancer Nursing*, **14**(2), 63–70.

Johns, C.C. (1989) Developing a philosophy for practice Part 1. *Nursing Practice*, **3**(1), 2–5.

Johns, C.C. (1991) The Burford Nursing Development Unit: holistic model of practice. *Journal of Advanced Nursing*, **16**(9), 1090–8.

McCaugherty, D. (1992) The Roper nursing model as an educational and research tool. *British Journal of Nursing*, **1**(9), 455–9.

Parkes, C.M. (1982) *Bereavement: Studies of Grief in Adult Life*, Tavistock, London.

Roper, N., Logan, W. and Tierney, A. (1983) *Using a Model for Nursing*, Churchill Livingstone, London.

FURTHER READING

Lamerton, R. (1980) *Care of the Dying*, Pelican, Harmondsworth.

Long, R. (1981) *Systematic Nursing Care*, Faber and Faber, London.

Nursing care in symptom management

4

Planning, implementation and evaluation

The documents used for the recording of nursing management are as varied as the treatment and care which are given. However, the aim should be clarity and simplicity, with the emphasis on the recording of ongoing assessment and evaluation.

Terminology also varies and the headings used in this chapter are only examples, among many in use. Many aspects of the nursing care of a dying patient are also applicable to the seriously ill patient who is likely to recover.

It is the 'special needs' associated with a number of common problems that will be considered here. Evaluation of the care given is implicit in the discussion and treatment may often have to be changed hourly rather than daily.

NAUSEA AND VOMITING

The patient feels ill, miserable and weak and there may be associated dizziness, headache and sweating. Constant retching may cause tenderness and bruising over the sternum.

Vomiting causes mental distress, since the patient feels that it is offensive to others and this lessens his or her own self-respect and dignity. Causes of nausea and vomiting in the dying patient are many and may include:

- acute infections, in particular of the urinary tract;
- hepatic metastases and uraemia;
- medications, in particular antibiotics and sometimes opiates (alcohol should not be taken if the patient is also receiving metronidazole);
- gastric irritation and intestinal obstruction;

- severe constipation;
- hypercalcaemia;
- raised intracranial pressure.

It must not be forgotten that the environment itself may be a cause of nausea and fear and anxiety often exacerbate the problem.

Aims of care

1. To identify the cause.
2. To help in the control of symptoms by administering prescribed antiemetic drugs or others appropriate for the cause.
3. To improve the patient's comfort.
4. To raise the patient's morale.

The symptoms may have been present for some time, and assurance must be given that immediate action will be taken to relieve the distress.

If a cause can be identified, such as severe constipation or a urinary tract infection, then the specific treatment should be commenced. Some causes of nausea and vomiting in the dying patient are difficult to deal with and therefore management may be symptomatic. Special attention to the mouth after vomiting is essential and mouthwashes are helpful, as is sponging of the face and hands. Soiled clothing and bedlinen should always be changed and vomit bowls emptied and returned. The latter, together with tissues, should be placed well within reach of the patient.

Fear and anxiety may exacerbate these symptoms and helping patients to talk about their fears and worries may help to relieve the situation. Even when vomiting is controlled, the fears that it could return are very real and the vomit bowl and tissues should remain at hand, but discreetly positioned.

Antiemetic medications and others

1. Antihistamines:
   - cyclizine 50 mg three times daily
   - promethazine 25 mg three times daily (but may cause drowsiness)
2. Butyrophenones:
   - haloperidol 0.5–1.5 mg three times a day. Prolonged use may cause extrapyramidal effects.
3. Phenothiazine:
   - prochlorperazine 5–10 mg 4-hourly or three times a day
   - methotrimeprazine 25 mg twice a day.

   These drugs have sedative and analgesic effects as well as being antiemetics. Prolonged or large doses of phenothiazine may cause twitching (dyskinesia) and sometimes a dry mouth. Both are usually relieved by lowering the dose.

4. Metoclopramide 5–10 mg three times a day. This drug accelerates gastric peristalsis and augments gastric emptying.
5. Domperidone 10 mg 4-hourly. This is a dopamine antagonist and affects gastric motility in a similar way to metoclopramide.
6. Chlorpromazine (by mouth 25–50 mg 3–4 times daily; by rectum 100 mg suppository 6–8-hourly). May be useful when hiccoughs are a problem and sedation is required.
7. Sodium clodronate by mouth 1.6 g daily or two divided doses. For hypercalcaemia due to malignancy.

This is not an exhaustive list and, depending on the cause of the nausea and vomiting, other drugs may be specifically effective. Many of the drugs can be given in combination and administered via a Graseby syringe driver, which may be the most effective and best tolerated route for the patient.

BOWEL PROBLEMS

Constipation

This symptom is a very real and common problem in the terminal stage of most illnesses. It leads to a most distressing and undignified situation for the patient.

The patient or relatives may mention the difficulty to the nurse or doctor, but a rectal examination should be performed as part of the admission assessment, as soon as it seems appropriate. The examination may reveal a state of impacted faeces.

Causes of constipation in the dying patient are the inevitable result of weakness and inactivity, diminished intake of food and fluid and the side effects of medication, especially opiates. Diarrhoea may accompany severe constipation, but is usually resolved when the hard faeces are removed. There may also be a mechanical bowel obstruction caused by a malignant growth.

Aims of care

1. To deal with the present condition by clearing the rectum and lower bowel.
2. To take appropriate measures to prevent recurrence of constipation, which can include regular administration of aperients, rectal suppositories or enemas.
3. To maintain hygiene.

4. To be aware of the patient's embarrassment or distress and to ensure privacy and help as needed.

It is the main aim of the nurse to try and prevent constipation in the dying patient and therefore the recording of when bowels are opened is an essential task. This will be maintained by discreet questioning and observation or by rectal examination on a regular basis. The patient's 'normal' routine should be determined, but as a result of illness this may no longer be relevant. Again it is essential that the patient understands this management.

The medication available is very varied, but a combination of a bowel stimulant and a faecal softener should be given on a regular basis. If constipation is severe or the patient very weak, then the combined treatment of glycerine and bisacodyl (Dulcolax) suppositories should result in less discomfort to the patient and a saving on nursing time.

An olive oil retention enema, given the previous night and followed in the morning by a phosphate enema, may be necessary when faeces are very hard.

Sometimes a manual removal of faeces may be the only possible action. Local anaesthetic lubricant such as Xylocaine can be used to lessen the discomfort. Midazolam 2 mg i.v. over 30 seconds may also be given as it combines a sedative effect with amnesia. Therefore the patient will have no memory of the procedure, should it have to be repeated.

Diarrhoea

Unless there is a specific pathological reason, true faecal incontinence is uncommon until the final hours, when weakness prevents control.

Causes of diarrhoea may include:

- medication – some antibiotics;
- radiotherapy;
- pancreatic tumours;
- anxiety and nervous tension.

Aims of care

1. To give appropriate treatment to control diarrhoea.
2. To maintain hygiene.
3. To preserve the patient's dignity.

Caring for a weak and ill patient suffering from diarrhoea requires very sensitive and skilful nursing. Help to reach the toilet or commode should be given promptly and the call bell must be within reach. Attention must be given to the care of the skin, in order to prevent excoriation.

Privacy must be maintained and efforts made to lessen unpleasant odours, by the use of deodorants. Incontinence pants and pads may be appropriate and may lessen the fear of 'accidents'. Anxiety should be recognized and if appropriate and acceptable, counselling should be given by a skilled person.

The following medications may be used:

- codeine phosphate, 15 mg three times daily;
- loperamide hydrochloride, 2 mg three times daily;
- domperidone, 10–20 mg 4–8-hourly;
- pancreatin preparations; Pancrex V is available when given with food for steatorrhoea;
- diazepam, 2–5 mg 3 times daily.

It is important to ensure that medications such as codeine phosphate are discontinued as soon as the diarrhoea ceases, so that subsequent constipation is avoided.

Stomata

Care of a patient with colostomy or other stoma will depend largely on how long the patient has had it and his or her ability to cope with it (or the ability of a member of the family who has been helping in the matter). A patient with a long-established stoma will have become used to a particular type of appliance and his or her own way of dealing with this and it is best to continue in the same way during the terminal illness. Obviously as the patient becomes weaker he or she may need help from nursing staff or family. Offering assistance as a patient loses control is always a sensitive step. Having a stoma is for many people a private affair and such matters as disposal of equipment may have been dealt with in a secret way, so the nurse needs to consider the patient's sensitivity here. The nurse should consult the patient as to his or her preferences in attending to the hygiene of the stoma. A nurse may have access to a nurse specialist, i.e. a stoma care nurse, if advice is needed.

Problems of abnormal stool consistency, soreness of surrounding mucosa and skin or malignant tissue in the actual stoma or surrounding area may be present. The many firms specializing in stoma care equipment are always pleased to help with information about types of equipment.

Sometimes a patient who has had an abdominoperineal resection of colon will have a troublesome discharge from the rectal stump. The administration of steroid suppositories and insertion of Proctofoam rectally often gives relief.

PROBLEMS WITH THE URINARY TRACT

Problems with the urinary tract can cause much distress to a dying patient, particularly incontinence and urinary infection. Urinary retention and frequency of micturition can both be due to intrapelvic tumours affecting the bladder or to spinal cord compression. Incontinence may occur for many reasons which include:

- medication (diuretics);
- infection (which may lead to confusion);
- neurological problems;
- urinary fistula;
- anxiety, weakness and lethargy;
- confusion;
- constipation (but this should not be a cause following admission assessment and ongoing management).

Aims of care

1. To preserve the patient's independence in using the lavatory or commode for as long as possible.
2. To take particular care with hygiene of the genital area.
3. To encourage sufficient fluids for as long as the patient is able to take them.
4. To be prepared to catheterize the patient, following careful assessment and explanation, in order to maintain comfort and dignity.
5. To administer drugs prescribed by the doctor which will alleviate symptoms.

For all patients in the terminal stage of illness it is most important that the nurse does everything possible to maintain continence. Assisting patients to the lavatory or ensuring a commode is within reach are important factors, as is privacy. Seat heights which can be adjusted or rails fixed beside the toilet or commode will maintain a further degree of independence.

In practice, bed pans are less often used, but urinals should be available. The call bell must be within reach. Catheterization may be a suitable option, but assessment should be thorough and patient choice and sometimes that of their family should be sought. It may well lessen the distress of incontinence, particularly when there is skin excoriation, oedema or a pressure sore in the sacral or genital area or when frequent moving adds to discomfort.

Alternatively, a uridom may be used for a man, but care must be taken to observe for soreness and that it does remain in position. Catheterization should not be withheld because of the risks of infection.

For some patients who have had long term catheterization there is a risk of septicaemia, following the manipulation involved in recatheterization (due to previously colonized bacteria, usually Gram negative, being transferred into the bloodstream).

It is therefore advisable that for these patients, and for those known to have a urinary tract infection prior to catheterization, antibiotic cover should be given. A single dose of gentamicin i.m. should be given one hour before the procedure, for which the suggested dose is:

- 60 mg for small patients
- 80 mg for those of average weight
- 100 mg for heavy patients.

In addition, if a urinary tract infection is present, oral antibiotics to which the infection is sensitive should be given for at least 48 hours. If there is doubt as to whether infection is present, or the MSU result is not available, then the use of gentamicin is recommended. However, for patients in terminal coma who become incontinent but are likely to die within a few days, antibiotics would not be necessary.

There is not usually a problem with drainage even when the patient's fluid intake is below average. Bladder washouts are not often required, but may be necessary if there are difficulties with drainage, as might occur with carcinoma of the bladder.

For the patient for whom catheterization is not acceptable, by choice or due to confusion or when the catheter becomes frequently blocked, then the use of pads may be a suitable option. There is a considerable range available and the selection may be made by choice, comfort, size and shape, absorbency and possibly cost.

Urinary infections

There are not uncommon in dying patients and the nurse must be aware that signs and symptoms may appear unrelated to the urinary tract, for instance vomiting, confusion or headache. An appropriate antibiotic is usually prescribed to relieve the painful and distressing symptoms. If painful urethral spasm is present, Urispas, 200 mg three times daily may be helpful.

PROBLEMS WITH NUTRITION AND FLUID INTAKE

With progressive weakness, patients with advanced terminal illness may become unable to take a normal diet or sufficient fluids. The nurse must recognize that this fact in itself often causes great anxiety to patients and in particular to their families.

There are several aspects to this problem, which are as follows.

1. There may be an obstructive lesion in the gastrointestinal tract (or upper respiratory tract) preventing the normal ingestion and passage of food and liquids. In the early stage of the disease, the patient with such a problem may have commenced artificial feeding by nasogastric tube or gastrostomy tube.
2. Anorexia eventually becomes a problem for all dying patients no matter what the particular disease. There may be some underlying factors contributing to the lack of appetite, for instance, certain types of therapy (e.g. cytotoxic drugs); nausea; constipation; gastrointestinal lesions; jaundice; uraemia; anxiety or depression; sore, dry or infected mouth; or inappropriate diet offered.

During the last 48 hours of life it is not unusual for the patient to become increasingly unable to take any nourishment by mouth, except sips of fluids, before lapsing into unconsciousness.

Helping the patient to eat and drink

In everyday life the average person in reasonable health enjoys meals and 'feels better' for them. There are psychological as well as physical reasons for this. Likewise, the patient who is terminally ill benefits from a balanced intake of food and fluids in the form of ordinary meals for as long as possible, even though the helpings of food will usually be small.

It must be stressed that, when encouraging the patient to eat and drink, it is important to remember that dietary preferences are very individual whether in health or in illness and so the approach must be in similar manner. The reasons for encouraging the patient to eat and drink are as follows.

1. Taking regular fluids, if necessary as small, frequent drinks, will help to keep the mouth moist and fresh and thus more comfortable. Fungal and other oral infections are common in the dying patient and some of the drugs in common use cause dryness of the mouth. Together with oral hygiene, frequent drinks will help to lessen the discomfort of these conditions. They will also prevent concentration of urine and lessen the risk of urinary infection.
2. Eating a certain amount of solid food, containing some roughage, helps to counteract constipation and, again, chewing of this food encourages salivation and a moist mouth. The risk of pressure sores with their attendant pain and discomfort is ever-present in the dying patient. Regular intake of protein helps to prevent this, in whatever food the patient can best assimilate.
3. While the patient remains alert, every effort should be made for his or

her life to be as normal and as pleasurable as possible. This includes making mealtimes enjoyable social occasions. Family involvement should be encouraged, especially if they are able to provide favourite snacks and drinks, and they are often appreciative of being invited to help.

Helping to maintain appetite

The aims of care are as follows.

1. Enabling choice. Involving the patient and family in choosing what is acceptable.
2. Flexibility of approach with regard to times of meals.
3. Carrying out any prescribed medical treatment that may improve the patient's appetite or any nursing measure which will alleviate a contributory cause of anorexia.

The first consideration is to control any distressing symptoms that are preventing the patient from wanting to eat or drink. Pain control is important, but above all is the relief of nausea and vomiting. It should be remembered that antiemetic drugs take a little while to become effective and a combination of drugs may be more effective still. A sore or unpleasant tasting mouth will also be a deterrent to the desire to eat. Dentures may have become ill-fitting as a result of continuing illness and wearing them may exacerbate the problem of a sore mouth or even be the cause.

The administration of small doses of steroids will usually have a stimulating effect on the appetite and this will be much appreciated by a patient if they have previously experienced a period of anorexia. If the appetite is improved, favourite foods may be enjoyed again (even jellied eels) and morale can be boosted. It should also be mentioned that patients who have been taking relatively large doses of steroids for a specific medical condition can develop an abnormal appetite, with constant craving for food during their terminal illness. Within all reasonable limits, such patients should be allowed what they wish.

Small amounts of alcohol are often enjoyed and, when taken as an apéritif, may also improve appetite and boost morale. The combination of alcohol and prescribed medication is not usually a problem in terminal illness. However, alcohol and metronidazole should not be taken together.

Presenting food and drink

Once the patient's appetite has been restored, small helpings of food at usual mealtimes are often enjoyed up to a day or two before death. This is more likely to happen if a detailed assessment has been made of the patient's food preferences and if the food is attractively presented and manageable. Too strict an adherence to previous dietary restrictions for medical reasons is now out of place. It is important to try and meet the patient's special needs which are part of their cultural or religious observances.

The patient should be assisted to a comfortable position, whether in bed or in a chair, and table heights should be appropriate. Fresh fruit will be more acceptable and enjoyable if it has been prepared in a manner which makes for easy handling and eating. It also helps to moisten the mouth.

The environment in which meals are taken should be as pleasant and relaxed as possible. Patients should not be hurried with their meals and this is especially important when help is required with feeding.

The nurse or carer should be encouraged to sit adjacent to the patient, on a similar level, when help with feeding is necessary. Feeder beakers may be acceptable to patients who find holding a cup difficult and who are concerned about spillage, thus prolonging independence a little longer. Gradually, the dying patient will only tolerate minimal amounts of food and it will be a challenge to the nurse to encourage fluids which are palatable and which will hydrate and nourish as far as possible.

Soups, commercial preparations such as Ensure Plus and Frebusan and ice cream milkshakes are often enjoyed, as are fizzy drinks and for many, the favourite cup of tea. Choice is paramount, as is providing that choice willingly at any time, be it day or night. Whilst a reasonable fluid intake is desirable for as long as possible, this will become increasingly difficult. In the period before unconsciousness occurs, sucking at flavoured ice lollies or on sponges dipped in fruit juice or taking tiny ice chips may be thirst-quenching and enjoyable. The nurse must be alert at all times to observe for changes in swallowing ability or alterations in the levels of consciousness.

The decision as to whether it is ethically correct to institute some form of artificial feeding in the terminal stages of illness is discussed in Chapter 14.

PROBLEMS INVOLVING THE SKIN AND MUCOUS MEMBRANE

The skin, being such a vital organ, will reflect many aspects of the patient's bodily and mental state and may be the cause of discomfort if not actual suffering. In assessing the condition of the skin the nurse may have observed abnormalities of colour:

- pallor – possibly due to anaemia or apprehension;
- jaundice – due to disease of the liver or biliary tract;
- cyanosis – due to cardiac or respiratory disease;

- cachexia – the typical greyish facial hue with gaunt cheeks commonly seen in patients with advanced cancer and accompanying other symptoms;
- petechiae – scattered bleeding of small blood vessels, abnormalities common in renal failure and blood dyscrasias

and of texture:

- dryness – due to dehydration;
- sweating – may be due to fever and fear;
- shiny, taut skin with underlying swelling – oedema;
- the puffy, moon face (Cushing's syndrome) which may accompany steroid drug therapy;
- pressure sores – these can occur in the terminal stage of any disease and range from small abrasions to deep cavities;
- widespread scratch marks – the patient's reaction to intense itching that causes much misery. The underlying cause may be obstructive jaundice or allergic reaction to drug therapy.

Pressure sores

Any patient in the terminal stage of an illness, irrespective of the particular disease, is at risk of developing pressure sores, as the body systems deteriorate, especially the vascular system. With an inefficient blood supply and diminished metabolic activity in the tissues it is not surprising that sores develop easily. There may be other factors contributing to the risk, such as emaciation or the presence of gross sacral and ankle oedema. Increasing weakness means that patients are less able to turn themselves in bed or to shift their position if sitting in a chair. Once the early signs of an incipient pressure sore appear, i.e. an unhealthy redness of the skin, tissue breakdown can proceed at an alarming rate until a large necrotic area becomes infected and causes sloughing to take place.

Fungating lesions

These are most common in breast cancer, but may occur in many other sites, such as lymph node metastases in neck or axilla. They may also occur in mucous membranes such as those in the vagina or rectum. Other situations in which fungating lesions may occur are in malignant melanoma and epithelioma of the skin.

Stomata

The patient may have an artificial opening onto the skin as a direct result of his or her present disease process, particularly in malignant disease or incidental to this. Colostomy and ileostomy are common; gastrostomy may also be present. These may be well managed or present problems of inflammation of skin and mucous membrane.

Aims of care

1. To give meticulous attention to the cleanliness of the skin.
2. To try to prevent pressure sores by relieving pressure on vulnerable areas and protecting the skin.
3. To relieve the pain and discomfort of lesions of the skin and mucous membranes by appropriate topical treatment and administration of other drugs, e.g. by the oral route.
4. If there is a problem of odour, to take steps to minimize this.

Care of the skin and general toilet

Washing the patient's skin should be carried out with due regard for personal preferences. Being immersed in a warm bath can be very relaxing and soothing and even a very ill patient can find this procedure pleasurable. In the bathroom, a soft appliance in the bath will help the thin patient. On the other hand, there should not be a relentless routine approach to giving the patient a bath either in bed or in the bathroom. Timing is important so that the patient does not feel exhausted. If an overall wash cannot be tolerated at a particular time, washing the face with special care of the eyes, the axillae and groins will help the patient feel fresh and comfortable.

Patients should be allowed to do as much for themselves as they wish, the nurse helping with areas of difficulty such as the feet and back and assisting with manicure of finger and toenails. Women patients and some male patients will appreciate the use of their favourite brand of talcum powder and perfume or aftershave. Care of the hair is vital in both sexes for comfort and appearance; this is something a relative who wishes to help can be asked to do if the patient cannot manage. A visit from the hairdresser when appropriate can be a great morale booster. Men should be helped to shave daily for the same reason.

Prevention of pressure sores

All patients should be assessed on admission and as frequently as necessary thereafter in order to ascertain their level of risk for skin breakdown. The condition of the skin should be noted on admission and then daily for signs of improvement or deterioration.

Nurses will be familiar with a range of assessment scales and will have evaluated their use in determining risk. In practice no one particular scale may be ideal for the terminally ill patient, but the simple Norton or the more complex Waterlow scales may be suitably adapted to assess the individual patient.

The terminally ill patient is at extreme risk of skin breakdown and many patients are admitted with pressure sores. Therefore, a detailed assessment will enable a care plan to be devised which will include preventative and therapeutic measures and which can be incorporated into the total plan of care.

It must be stressed that assessment of mobility and the planning for safe handling and lifting should be incorporated into care for the prevention and/or treatment of pressure sores. More on this is given in the section on mobility.

The patient should be encouraged to be out of bed for as much of the day as he or she feels able; this activity will, of course, gradually come to an end. Once the patient needs to be in bed all the time, regular turning and attention to all pressure areas must be carried out meticulously, which will include maintaining cleanliness of the skin and using an appropriate barrier cream if considered helpful.

As with other patients at particular risk, a suitable pressure relieving aid may be helpful. These may include pressure relieving mattresses or padding systems, such as:

- Spenco mattresses and similar;
- large cell ripple mattresses;
- air-wave support systems (Pegasus).

The most suitable aid will be determined following assessment of the individual patient's needs. For example, the priority might be preventative for a frail elderly patient or a heavy patient becoming more disabled as a result of spinal cord compression or a patient with as yet ill-controlled pain and existing pressure sores. (We have found that a 'net turning' bed has been useful and comfortable for heavy patients with spinal cord compression.)

It should be remembered that the patient sitting in a chair, no less than the patient in bed, needs to have regular changes of position and a pressure-relieving aid. The use of an indwelling catheter for the dying patient who is incontinent of urine will prevent maceration of the skin and lessen the risk of pressure sores developing.

Wounds

Sometimes the dying patient will have a wound varying from a healing postoperative one to a large ulcerated lesion that includes pressure sores. Patients with cancer may have external growths that require attention. These will vary from a dry undressed area to a large, discharging open wound which is ulcerated and with an offensive odour. Such a wound may be encroaching on blood vessels, which gives rise to a risk of slight or severe bleeding. Malignant growths may also have destroyed the bony structure of the face and the patient may find the wearing of sunglasses helpful. These wounds often cause much embarrassment especially if they are offensive. Occasionally a patient may deny their existence.

Nursing staff should be very sensitive to such problems and must be careful to show no signs of repugnance when dealing with the dressings. Following assessment, it may seem appropriate to request the specialist tissue viability nurse to visit and offer advice.

Ulcerated or discharging wounds will require cleansing and a suitable dressing and it might be prudent for a wound swab to be taken. As a result, appropriate antibiotics may be prescribed. Occasionally it may be necessary for patients to be nursed in isolation or a patient may request a single room because of the distress their wound causes. However, care must be taken to ensure that the isolation is as minimal as possible and that the wound does not lessen close contact.

Management of wounds is very varied and many dressing materials are available. Management should also include consideration of the patient's nutritional intake and if possible food supplements are encouraged.

Dressing suggestions:

1. Cavities, fistulae or sinuses need to be well cleansed and a syringe or catheter can be used for irrigation.
2. When drainage from a wound or fistula is profuse, a colostomy bag may be fitted, which will help to reduce the frequency of dressing changes and minimize soiling of clothes and odour. It may also help to maintain the integrity of the surrounding skin.
3. The use of charcoal dressing pads or the deodorant Nilodor may help to reduce offensive odour. Alternatively, metronidazole 400 mg 8-hourly given orally or used as a gel and combined with the dressing (although very costly) may lessen the odour of a fungating wound.
4. Wounds liable to bleed may benefit from the use of the Kaltostat (calcium alginate) range. If severe bleeding is considered likely, then the patient should have had an adrenaline 1 in 1000 solution prescribed and also sedation, so that the treatment can be administered immediately if the condition arises. It is a most alarming situation and as calm an atmosphere as possible should be maintained. The use of a red blanket will also be required.
5. If dressing changes are likely to cause increased pain, then suitable additional analgesia should be given at an appropriate time beforehand. Inhalational patient controlled analgesia (Entonox) may also be used.
6. Cleansing agents/desloughing agents. As with all aspects of care,

assessment of the wound should take place in order to plan management. Nurses should be aware of recent research in regard to many 'traditional' cleansing lotions, for example Morgan (1992). Antiseptic lotions such as cetrimide may have a toxic effect on wound healing.

Sensitization may occur with chlorhexidine. Chlorinated solutions such as Eusol may delay healing, be irritant and cause localized oedema and the use of Eusol is not now advised. It is likely that sodium chloride is just as effective, unless the wound is heavily infected. Other alternatives to chlorinated solutions are modern products such as:

- hydrocolloids – Granuflux paste;
- alginates – Sorbsan;
- Debrisan beads or paste.

Intense itching

If severe, this can cause great distress and misery to the dying patient, whose threshold of tolerance is likely to be low. The nurse will be asked to apply an appropriate topical application according to the cause of the irritation. Oral medication may also be prescribed. Fungal infections are common, especially in the inguinal and perianal regions, and pruritus often accompanies jaundice and uraemia. It should not be forgotten that itching could be drug-induced.

Medication which may be of use includes:

- Canesten pessaries/cream for vaginal thrush;
- antihistamines – the sedative effect may be helpful;
- calamine lotion;
- emollients used in the bath may be helpful for very dry skin.

Oedema

There may be many causes of generalized oedema in the terminally ill patient. Localized oedema may result in massive enlargement of a limb, especially of an arm in women patients following radical mastectomy.

This is now more often seen in elderly patients, as such surgery is less often performed today. The physiotherapist may be asked to assess the patient in order to see if bandaging of the limb or the use of pressure-pumping apparatus would be helpful. Similar treatment may be appropriate for oedema of the legs. Other means to aid comfort, such as the judicious use of cushions and foot stools to support limbs, should be tried.

The nurse may be asked to assist the doctor in removing ascitic fluid from a dying patient if this is causing distress because of distension or breathlessness.

Tracheostomy

It is not uncommon for the nurse to care for a terminally ill patient who has a tracheostomy, usually performed for a malignant condition. The actual care of the tracheostomy site will be the same as for other patients, but dying patients will need special understanding regarding their need for communication as they become weaker. If they have been dealing with the tracheostomy themselves they may feel anxious about having to leave this to a nurse whom they do not know when admitted to a hospital, if they are too weak to continue. Having one or two nurses only to deal with this will inspire confidence as they get to know the patient and their needs. There may be a member of the family who has become skilled in the matter and should be consulted about any details of information that will be helpful; indeed, he or she should be allowed to continue to help with the procedure if desired.

PROBLEMS ASSOCIATED WITH MOBILITY

Many dying patients have few such problems until the last few days of their illness, when increasing weakness overtakes them. Other patients may become virtually immobile for many weeks or months during the terminal stage of their illness. This may be as a direct result of neurological, cardiovascular or muscular disorders or as a signal to certain forms of malignant disease – for example, cord compression due to metastatic spread from cancer of the prostate gland or breast or motor neurone disease.

Some patients may indeed have had years of immobility due to a chronic neurological disease, such as multiple sclerosis, so that the terminal stage is simply a continuation of the problem.

Dangers of immobility are similar at any stage of an illness, notably: pressure sores; pneumonia; muscle wasting; and joint contractures. Apart from these potential dangers, the patient who is unable to move without help will often become physically uncomfortable and psychologically frustrated.

Aims of care

1. To organize a regular programme of changing the patient's position whether in bed or sitting in a chair.
2. To ensure that all limbs are gently exercised and placed in anatomically correct positions.

3. To avoid overtiring the patient in any therapeutic endeavour.
4. To cooperate with the physiotherapist in his or her efforts for the patient's comfort.
5. To control any symptoms which are restricting mobility.

It is therefore essential that assessments of mobility and of 'handling risk factors' are included in the patient's admission assessment and as often thereafter as their condition warrants. The nursing care plan, whatever its design, must include an action plan in respect of handling. This should include the patient's abilities and inabilities and how lifting and handling are to be carried out. All staff should be competent in lifting techniques and feel confident in the use of lifting aids. These may include hoists and lifting straps. If nursing staff are confident, then it will help to encourage patients who, understandably, are often reluctant to be 'hoisted'.

PROBLEMS ASSOCIATED WITH MOUTH CARE

Good mouth care is important in all areas of nursing and in addition there are extra factors that demand close observation and attention when patients are dying. This section briefly discusses two main subject areas:

1. The reasons why mouth care may be of special importance in terminal illness.
2. The components of mouth care for such patients.

Mouth deterioration is not inevitable in the dying patient. Perhaps this is the most important reason for giving the correct care, since mouths may then be kept in a good condition. It has been noted that they may be restored even in the face of rapid general deterioration.

Problems involving the mouth

Poor mouths have bad physical and psychological effects. A dry mouth will often feel unpleasant and result in difficulty with eating. When a patient knows that his or her mouth is not quite right there is fear of halitosis and consequent withdrawal from others. All these situations diminish the quality of life. Terminally ill patients are often elderly and have denture problems. Loss of weight may lead to dentures fitting badly and rubbing may produce open sores that may proceed to infection because the wearing of dentures occludes air from oral surfaces. Patients may have been deteriorating over a long period during which weakness has reduced their ability to care for their mouths. In their last days patients may lack full consciousness and the ability to complain of a distressing mouth condition. They may also be unable to experience the sensations that would warn of trouble. Other reasons why mouth care is especially important in dying patients are as follows.

1. Terminally ill patients have often had inadequate diets for long periods if they have been experiencing nausea and vomiting for some time or have been living alone and unable to make the effort to obtain a balanced diet. Other patients, for instance those having steroids, tend to assuage their hunger with excessive carbohydrate intake. Unless the debris is removed adequately there can be a very rapid deterioration of the gingiva, increasing greatly the patient's general misery.
2. Very sick patients are often reluctant to eat and drink. One of the effects is that the salivary glands are then not stimulated to function. This results in poor clearance of the mouth and the debris left acts as a focus of infection.
3. Many drugs affect the mouth, including those previously given to terminally ill patients. Examples are immunosuppressive agents, corticosteroids and antibiotics and also antidepressants.

Aims of care

1. To prevent mouth deterioration by regular observation and the choice of the most suitable cleansing agents.
2. To maintain a clean, comfortable mouth with the patient's cooperation.
3. To report any abnormality immediately so that the appropriate treatment may be instituted without delay.

Regular observations of the whole mouth

This should be daily for patients whose condition is weak and deteriorating. It is often a practice to observe the tongue alone but candida infection and other disorders can affect all the oral mucosae. The most natural and least disturbing time for this inspection is when the patient is normally receiving mouth care and removing dentures. Many patients are so weak or nauseous that denture removal is a real effort.

Encouragement towards self-help

Whenever possible, mouth care is best undertaken by the patient, with assistance if necessary to provide help and confidence. The patient alone will know the tender spots and those where pressure would cause retching. Those who have difficulty swallowing or breathing may find mouth care a very frightening procedure. If they can be gently helped in an unhurried way to control the process then confidence will be gained.

Care tailored to the needs of the individual

Assessment and planning are necessary and this includes both the timing and the process of care. It may be sufficient for the ambulant patient with a reasonable appetite to clean and refresh their mouth after meals; the unconscious patient, particularly the mouth breather, will require 2-hourly attention. This should be given when lying on his or her side, great care being taken that he or she does not aspirate any fluid. Other patients who have dry mouths and anorexia have been found to benefit from oral care before meals so that salivary glands and appetite are stimulated.

It is likely that the regularity and the process of care, rather than the agents used, are most effective. The use of gloves is recommended for care other than the simple use of toothbrush and paste and certainly for denture cleaning (Clarke, 1993).

Removing debris

Small, soft toothbrushes have been found to be effective for removing debris from all surfaces of the teeth. The use of foam covered sticks (sponges) is also accepted and tolerated by many patients, but their use may be less effective.

Placing a half tablet of vitamin C on the tongue and allowing it to dissolve will clean debris and is well tolerated by many patients. The effervescent action on the oral mucosa is unlikely to have the potentially damaging effect of sodium bicarbonate or hydrogen peroxide. There is also evidence to show that a mixture of mouthwash, ice chips and tap water applied to the tissues might reduce the surface tension and penetrate the mucous barrier, stimulate the blood flow and, through friction, remove the remaining sordes which could then be rinsed out with the mixture.

Moistening, softening, freshening, stimulating

Mouthwashes moisten and soften the tissues although their refreshing effect is thought to be very transient. Mild commercial mouthwashes may be used or normal saline. Redoxan mouthwashes have been found to be useful when patients have a fear of swallowing other types. Research indicates that chlorhexidine (Corsodyl) has an antiplaque effect. Fruit juices may also be effective in mouth care, in addition to providing fluids, as they moisten, refresh and stimulate. Lemon stimulates the salivary glands, but care must be taken to avoid overfrequent use, as there may be a 'reflex exhaustion' effect. The use of lemon swabs, especially for a very weak patient, may be an acceptable and tolerated way of moistening the mouth.

Similarly the use of the foam sponges dipped in fruit juice is helpful in giving mouth care or a small amount of fluid to the dying patient.

Care of the lips

Dryness can soon develop in very painful cracks that provide sites for candida infection. Lips may be cleansed gently with saline swabs and Vaseline or lip salves applied.

Care of dentures

Dentures should be cleaned separately and care must be taken to avoid scratching the surface by the use of an abrasive substances. Hot water could cause them to warp and they should not be left to dry (Clarke, 1993). For the debilitated patient whose illness has caused loss of weight and a change in shape of the oral structure, the dentures may no longer fit comfortably and may indeed cause friction. The nurse must be observant for such problems.

Reporting abnormalities

All abnormalities must be reported as soon as possible. For the terminally ill and debilitated patient, the smallest oral sore can cause great distress and they are prone to candida infections. A variety of antifungal medications is available and can be used in a local or systemic approach. Such oral medications must be allowed to come into contact with all oral surfaces. Therefore application should be made to dentures separately.

RESPIRATORY PROBLEMS

There are a number of diseases in which symptoms related to the respiratory tract may become very distressing to the patient during the terminal stage of the illness. The commonest symptoms are cough; excessive, sometimes purulent or bloodstained sputum; dyspnoea; haemoptysis; and chest pain.

Causes of dyspnoea in a dying patient may be the result of a chronic condition such as asthma, chronic bronchitis or congestive cardiac failure or of a malignant tumour infiltrating the lungs and other parts of the respiratory tract.

Pneumonia is common in the terminal stage of many illnesses. Fear or anxiety may produce dyspnoea which itself leads to further tension and thus a vicious circle of cause and effect. Cough is another problem that may be present in association with dyspnoea and sometimes from the same cause.

Aims of care

1. To provide the most comfortable physical position to ease the patient's dyspnoea or cough.
2. To administer drugs and assist with other forms of treatment prescribed by the doctor.
3. To cooperate with the physiotherapist if required.
4. To try to lessen emotional tension that may be aggravating the dyspnoea.

General principles of care

Positioning the patient

Most patients with respiratory problems are more comfortable when sitting upright. They will need plenty of pillows and some form of backrest. Some patients are more at ease sitting in an armchair than in bed and may insist on doing so for much of the time until they lose consciousness.

Mouth care

The nurse should remember that respiratory symptoms are often accompanied by a dry and unpleasant tasting mouth, so mouth care becomes even more important.

Fear and anxiety

Some respiratory symptoms arouse great fear in the patient and in the family too. The dyspnoeic patient feels he may be suffocating and the panic induced will further increase the problem and so a vicious circle is set up. Haemoptysis is very frightening and there may have been several episodes prior to a catastrophic one occurring at the time of death.

Special measures

Cough

This may be dry and unproductive and is very exhausting for the patient. A simple linctus in hot water often seems to offer relief. The productive cough with mucopurulent sputum is also exhausting. A short course of broad spectrum antibiotics may give considerable relief, as will gentle physiotherapy.

The administration of small doses of opioids (Oramorph) may also achieve good relief.

Dyspnoea

Dyspnoea is a terrifying symptom. 'The sensation of being unable to breath adequately will generate tremendous fear and panic" (Finlay, 1991). It is vital to try to determine the underlying cause and to establish to what degree fear and anxiety (especially that of dying) are exacerbating the symptom. Patients should not be left alone and subdued lighting at the bedside at night should be provided.

The nurse's understanding of the causes of dyspnoea and in particular the psychological aspects should enable a confident, reassuring and gentle manner, which is important when caring for patients. Allowing the patient to feel cool air on the face may be comforting and can be achieved by positioning them near an open window or perhaps more readily with a carefully positioned electric fan. The administration of oxygen for short periods may also be beneficial, but more benefit may be achieved by the nurse sitting beside the patient and giving confident reassurance.

Relaxation and therefore relief may also be achieved by alternative therapies. Aromatherapy, reflexology and the playing of relaxing music have been used with very positive results.

Drugs used will be related to the cause of the dyspnoea, for instance diuretics in the case of pulmonary oedema. The slowing down of the respiratory drive can be achieved by the use of opioids in a nebulized form. The dose can be titrated upwards in very small amounts until the severe dyspnoea is relieved. The dose will be in addition to that being given regularly for pain relief. Occasionally when there is a large pleural effusion, relief will be obtained by aspiration of the fluid. Similarly, consideration may be given to whether palliative radiation would be effective.

Haemoptysis

The patient may have had previous warning haemorrhages and if at all possible, this should have been elicited during admission assessment. Day and night staff should be informed as to the possibility of a major haemorrhage and therefore will be as prepared as possible. Relatives, too, should be given a gentle warning, but trying not to alarm them excessively.

Red towels and blankets should be available to spread over the bed, the idea being to lessen the frightening effect of blood loss. Medication should have previously been ordered, so that there will be little delay when the need arises to achieve rapid sedation. This can be achieved by opiates, diazepam or midazolam given by injection. Diazepam can also be given as a rectal preparation (Stesolid), if it is felt safe to turn the patient. Suction apparatus should be ready and close by. Blood transfusion is probably not appropriate at this time.

Severe haemoptysis is frightening and is a difficult situation for staff, who may long to take more active measures. However, the aim must be to enable the patient to die peacefully without 'busy' heroic measures. A member of staff must be at the bedside to hold the patient's hand or to support relatives if they are present. The relatives, if present, will need particular support and assurance about the manner of the patient's dying. The effect of this severe event on other patients must also be considered and reassurance may be necessary. Staff, too, must be allowed time to reflect and talk over this particular patient's manner of dying.

CONFUSION

Nurses may often have to care for a dying patient who is confused and it is not always easy to establish the cause. Again, assessment involving all staff and the patient and family is essential. But before assuming that the patient's problem is confusion, do take care to ascertain that it is not due to language comprehension and speech difficulties or cultural differences or even hearing deficit.

Confusion may well be caused by a combination of problems and it should not be forgotten that sometimes an episode of restlessness may precede confusion. The restlessness may be due to physical causes (such as urinary retention), anxiety or a combination of both.

Causes of confusion may be as follows.

- Known cerebrovascular disease.
- Cerebral metastases.
- Side effects of medication such as amitriptyline or carbamazepine.
- The sudden withdrawal of benzodiazepines or alcohol.
- Constipation, especially in the elderly.
- Metabolic upset such as hypercalcaemia or uraemia.
- Acute infections, urinary or respiratory.
- Uncontrolled pain.
- Emotional distress.
- The effect of a change in the environment, especially at night.

The confusion experienced is very distressing not only for the patient but especially for the family and relatives. It is also a problem for nursing staff and other patients. For the family, the memories of their loved one dying in such a distressed state can be very disturbing. Assessment involving the family or friends may help to elicit the previous mental state of the patient and whether previous life events might be relevant.

It is important to try and establish causes as the treatment of an acute infection by antibiotics or the relief of constipation can make such an improvement, as may the reduction of hypercalcaemia.

The patient will require gentle handling in a calm manner and there should be no attempt to argue if they appear hallucinated. The use of a side room is of very debatable value, but may need to be considered. The use of sedation is usually necessary and should not be equated with failure. However, relatives and staff must have adequate explanation as to why it is being given.

Drugs which may prove helpful, especially with the elderly, include haloperidol and Melleril. Nurses should be aware of the possibility of increased confusion after long term use of these drugs in some patients, especially those with diminished renal or hepatic function.

PSYCHOLOGICAL AND SPIRITUAL PROBLEMS

Dying patients now facing their own deaths may be consciously working out their beliefs for the first time. This may be with knowledge of a faith which has felt secure and sure until now or without belief or a philosophy of life and death. It may, however, become a time of crisis as they struggle to come to terms with their God who now seems to have abandoned them or as they grasp for some lifeline in their despair.

The individual who feels that God has abandoned them may have lived their life obeying a ‘God of rules’, but have failed to find or develop a personal relationship with God.

For carers it is a time of extreme importance, when they are doing their best for this unique individual, respecting and valuing their every part, be it body, mind or spirit, as they come to the end of life’s journey. It may be, too, that at this time, the carers themselves may experience a questioning of their own beliefs.

As Alun Jones (1993) writes, ‘Carers need the provision of a safe environment in which to explore, when caring for a dying patient’.

Psychological needs of the dying patient

The work of Elisabeth Kübler-Ross in enhancing awareness and understanding of patients’ responses to their dying process has been mentioned in other chapters. The role of the nurse in helping and supporting the patient in the light of this and other research will now be considered. As long as consciousness remains, powerful emotions will affect the patient's attitude and the degree of suffering or discomfort that he or she experiences. In their observation and assessment of this emotional state, nurses play a vital role in relieving the effect of painful emotions and involving the family and other colleagues in these efforts.

The first priority is for nurses to establish a relationship of trust with the patient. This will not develop if they give an impression of wanting to hurry away on every occasion and avoiding any real contact. By getting to know the patient they will have an awareness of the patient's emotional state which, of course, can change from day to day. Personality, family attitudes and the patient's physical condition are among the factors that will influence emotions and vice versa. The main emotional problems for which the patient needs help will now be discussed in outline and developed in subsequent chapters.

Fear

A fear of how the final phase of dying will occur is common and may be linked with anticipation of certain intolerable physical events such as choking to death. If patients can voice their fears to doctors and nurses, so that assurance can be given that these are unfounded, much relief will be given. Fear of the mystery of death and uncertainty as to an afterlife may be helped by offering the services of a minister of religion and this is discussed later.

Loneliness

This is sometimes linked with fear if patients feel there is no-one to whom they can turn to share the burden by listening to their problems. Nurses should be aware that patients can still feel lonely in a ward with other patients. Even if staff are busy, a smile and a pause to ask if that patient needs anything will reinforce a sense of personal care. Close physical contact with a loved one should not be denied, be it the holding of a hand, affectionate embrace or cuddle. Companionship or suitable diversionary activity helps to dispel loneliness, but we must be alert for the patient who prefers to lie or sit quietly alone or who is becoming overtired by too much activity.

Anxiety

The patient may tend to be of an anxious disposition already and the facts of dying can produce many particular anxieties such as worries about finance and family well-being and uncertainty about the prognosis of the illness. The nurse can play an important role in enlisting the help of other colleagues such as the social worker. To help the patient who becomes excessively anxious and agitated, drugs may be prescribed such as diazepam 2–5 mg twice or three times a day.

If dying patients are receiving care in an institution, they may express a great longing to see their homes again and become restless and anxious. Even if the patients are weak, it may be justifiable to meet this request and arrange for them to be taken home for a short visit. It is found that patients are often remarkably peaceful once they have achieved what they probably know is a last farewell to their homes.

Sadness

It is understandable that dying patients, who have insight into their condition, experience sadness at the impending loss of their life and all that they value, including those they love. There is no easy remedy to prescribe for this natural reaction, but if the care given by all the caring team is of a high quality, patients will at least be relieved of distressing symptoms that interfere with progress towards acceptance of their coming death. Where there are close family relationships and both patient and family have reached acceptance together, the remaining span of life can take on a new and precious quality. Talking to patients about the past may help to reinforce their self-esteem by showing that they are still an individual of value.

When admission time before death is extremely short, it is difficult to build that relationship of trust and support with patients and their families. In the time left, physical care often seems to take precedence, but every effort must be made to recognize the fears, anxieties and unresolved guilt and conflict that may exist.

Carr (1982) writes of the 'common fears of dying patients, which include fear of loneliness and dying alone', but goes on to speak of how nurses can help them to work through the fears and so achieve a dignified and peaceful death.

Depression

It is not always easy to distinguish sadness from depression, but it is important to treat the latter before it becomes severe and very distressing. The observations of the nurse will be vital, as the patient may assume a mask when the doctor visits and the true state of affairs can be missed at first. A psychiatrist or clinical psychologist may be asked to see the patient and antidepressant drugs will be prescribed. The timing is important, as these drugs do not usually have any significant effect until the patient has been taking them for about a week; this is a long time in terms of many terminal illness. One example of a useful drug is lofepramine 140–210 mg daily in two or three divided doses.

Depression may be one cause of insomnia, although of course there are many others. The nurse will often be involved in trying to help a patient to sleep, first by investigating the possible causes. There can be a number of physical causes or simple environmental problems such as noise or overheating of the ward or room. Specific remedies should be tried first, including sitting with the patient and quietly discussing a possible solution with him or her. Eventually, some patients will need sedation with drugs such as:

- temazepam 10–30 mg at night;
- choral hydrate 0.5 1 g at night (well mixed with fluid) may be useful for the elderly;
- Heminevrin (chlormethiazole) 1 2 capsules at night; may be useful if alcohol intake has been an earlier problem.

Weakness and tiredness

These are symptoms which are associated with the lethargy of terminal illness but may also accompany anxiety and depression. The administration of steroids such as Dexamethasone 2–6 mg daily is often helpful as it may provide a feeling of well-being, as well as stimulating an interest in food.

Cognitive function

Some dying patients appear to retain all their intellectual powers to the end. In others they begin to fail, the extent varying with the individual. The patient is less able to concentrate and cannot cope with activities such as reading or writing. Decision making becomes difficult and conversation limited to monosyllables. Some of these problems may be due directly to increasing physical weakness or the effects of drugs. Memory may be retained up to the end, even though the patient may not be able to demonstrate this verbally. The nurse may observe that the patient is restless and anxious about some unfinished business that they desire to complete before it is too late. For the patient's peace of mind and for the future well-being of their family it is important that the patient has put their financial affairs in order and has made a will. The nurse may be asked by the patient or family to help in this matter (see further details in Chapter 8). The tenacity to live to fulfil important events may be extraordinarily strong even in extreme weakness. Such examples as experiencing the happiness of seeing the first grandchild or a special wedding anniversary of the patient and spouse – literally hanging on to life by a thread to achieve the highlight of happiness – are common.

The role of religion

Religion has provided a visible framework of support and guidance to human beings in their endeavour to lead a good life and prepare for a life after death from the beginning of recorded history and beyond. This rests in a belief in the immortality of the human spirit and the existence of a higher power, namely the deity or sometimes more than one deity.

Death is usually seen as a gateway to an eternal life of perfect happiness. These spiritual beliefs, presented here in a simplistic way, have been of great solace to many dying people, although it is said that in Western society their numbers are declining. In Chapter 13 some details are given regarding the role of ministers of various religions in the spiritual care of patients and their families and how the nurse can assist in bringing this service to his or her patients.

Many people will say that they believe in God and some kind of an afterlife, without belonging to a particular religious faith. Others say that they believe that death is the end of the human person. Whatever their own attitudes, nurses should ask such patients if there is anything that they would find helpful if they do not wish to have religious facilities. They may like to read, or have read to them, words from the world's great philosophers or religious leaders, including the Psalms or words from the Christian gospels or books of other world religions. In some hospices, short prayers are said in the wards at the beginning and end of each day. Comments are often made by patients that they have found this custom a comfort to them. However, it would be intrusive to subject a patient to formal religious services in ward or chapel unless they wished to be present.

It should be remembered that in many religions certain physical actions and material objects used as symbols are very important to the believer and should be respected. Some examples nurses may meet are described in Chapters 6 and 13.

The reality of suffering

'Pain' is sometimes used synonymously with 'suffering', but perhaps the latter word is more vivid in summarizing the total condition of the dying patient that the nurse with other carers is seeking to mitigate. It encompasses all the distressing symptoms of mind and body described in this book and the close interaction between physical and psychological factors.

Suffering is a reality of life and always has been. It denotes something more than minor discomforts and, indeed, may be so devastating as to be described as intense, agonizing or intolerable. Through modern mass media, people are daily exposed to suffering on a global scale, some of it manmade but some natural. It provokes such question as 'Why does this happen to innocent people?'; 'If there is a God, why does He allow this?' Suffering through illness and dying also provokes these questions and the additional one, 'Why me?'. Many philosophers and theologians have attempted to find answers to these and similar questions and the wisest will say that there are no complete answers.

Some people profess that there is no meaning at all and would agree with Ernest Hemingway that 'Life is just a dirty trick, from nothingness to nothingness'. Others search for meaning and find this gradually through a lifetime of experience. Viktar Frankl (1963) wrote, after searing experiences in a concentration camp:

> If there is a meaning in life at all, then there must be a meaning in suffering. Suffering is an ineradicable part of life, even as fate and death. Without suffering and human death, life cannot be complete.

Those who have witnessed beauty, love and heroism demonstrated by suffering human individuals would agree with him. Those with a strong religious faith will find support to bear suffering in themselves and others, particularly if they believe in a loving God and an afterlife free from suffering. This does not exclude, at times of crisis, moments of doubt and anger with God and one's fellow humans.

The nurse and suffering

Nurses will feel more confident and comfortable in responding to questions from dying patients in bewilderment, anguish and anger at their suffering if they have worked through their own beliefs and have some knowledge of the patient's religious faith if they profess one (Chapter 13).

To be present and listening in sympathetic silence, or giving the quiet answer 'I think I would be feeling angry, too, in your position' is more valuable than attempting any theological or philosophical answer – even if one felt adequate to do so. There are now ample means to reduce physical pain in the dying patient so that this may become virtually non-existent and in turn will leave the patient less fearful and anxious.

However, the sufferings of the family may be far greater than the patient's, both in their anticipatory grieving and subsequent bereavement. Parkes (1975) found this to be more common in such instances as the loss of young children or where the bereaved person has other stresses both in present life and in the past. Again, the nurse in frequent contact with the family can share in carrying the burden of family suffering by empathetic listening as above and by cooperating with other caregivers who bring special skills to the bereaved individuals or families. These skills are described in a number of other chapters in this book.

Finally, since the nurse is brought into close contact with suffering in the realm of dying and bereaved people, it is not surprising that there is a considerable element of stress in these caregiving situations and that the nurse him or herself needs support (Chapter 13).

Acknowledgements

We would like to express our gratitude to Noreen Brogan, Staff Nurse at St Joseph's Hospice, and acknowledge the previous work of:

Beryl Munns – Problems associated with mouth care
Joy Robbins – Psychological and spiritual problems
Sister Catherine Egan – Nutrition and food intake
Bernadette Ross – Respiratory problems
Sister Helena McGilly

REFERENCES

Carr, A.T. (1982) Dying and bereavement, in *Psychology for Nurses and Health Visitors*, (ed. J. Hall), Macmillan, Basingstoke, pp. 217–38.

Clarke, G. (1993) Mouth care and the hospitalized patient. *British Journal of Nursing*, **2**(4), 225–7.

Finlay, I. The management of other frequently encountered symptoms, in *Palliative Care for People with Cancer*, (eds J. Penson and R. Fisher), Edward Arnold, London, pp. 54–76.

Frankl, V.E. (1963) *Man's Search for Meaning*, Pocket Books, New York.

Jones, A. (1993) A first step in effective communication. *Professional Nurse*, **8**(8), 501–5.

Morgan, D. (1992) *Wound Cleansing Agents*, Educational Leaflet No. 10, Wound Care Society.

Parkes, C.M. (1975) *Bereavement – Studies of Grief in Adult Life*, Penguin, Harmondsworth.

FURTHER READING

Ainsworth-Smith, I. and Speck, P. (1982) *Letting Go – Caring for the Dying and Bereaved*, SPCK, London.

Black, I. (1992) Terminal restlessness in patients with advanced malignant disease. *Journal of Palliative Medicine*, **6**(4), 293–8.

Bliss, M. and Thomas, J. (1993) An investigative approach into alternating pressure supports. *Professional Nurse*, **8**(9), 437–44.

Bjurbrant-Birgersson, A.M., Hammer, V., Widefors, G., Hallberg, I. and Athlin, E. (1993) Elderly women's feelings about being urinary incontinent and being helped by nurses to change napkins. *Journal of Clinical Nursing*, **2**(3), 165–71.

Centre for Medical Education (1992) *Helpful Essential Links to Palliative Care*, University of Dundee/Cancer Relief Macmillan Fund.

Collet, J. (1991) *Nutrition and Wound Healing*, Educational Leaflet No. 7, Wound Care Society.
Commission of the European Communities Directive (1990) *Minimum Health and Safety Requirements for the Manual Handling of Loads, Where There is a Risk of Back Injury*, CECD, Brussels.
Dealey, C. (1993) Pressure sores – result of bad nursing? *British Journal of Nursing*, **1**(15), 748.
Dealey, C. (1993) Role of hydrocolloids in wound management. *British Journal of Nursing*, **1**(7), 358–65.
Fawcett, H. (1993) Interpreting a moral right – ethical dilemmas in nutritional support for the terminally ill. *Professional Nurse*, **8**(6), 380–3.
Hanham, S. (1990) Management of constipation. *Nursing*, **4**(17), 28–31.
Health Service Advisory Committee (1992) *Guidance on Manual Handling of Loads in the Health Service*, HSAC, London.
Heals, D. (1993) A key to well-being: oral hygiene in patients with advanced cancer. *Professional Nurse*, **8**(6), 391–8.
House, N. (1992) The hydration question – hydration or dehydration of terminally ill patients? *Professional Nurse*, **8**(1), 44–8.
House, N. (1993) Helping to reach an understanding – palliative care for people from ethnic minority groups. *Professional Nurse*, **8**(5), 329–32.
Larcombe, J. (1993) Too heavy to handle. *Nursing Times*, **89**(40), 46–50.
Lewis, C.S. (1957) *The Problem of Pain*, Fontana, London.
Lichter, I. (1990) Weakness in terminal care. *Journal of Palliative Medicine*, **4**(2), 73–80.
Lichter, I. (1991) Some psychological causes of distress in the terminally ill. *Journal of Palliative Medicine*, **5**(2), 138–46.
Lowthian, P. (1993) Acute patient care: pressure areas. *British Journal of Nursing*, **2**(9), 449–56.
McNamara, P., Minton, M. and Twycross, R. (1991) Use of midazolam in palliative care. *Palliative Medicine*, **5**(3), 244–9.
Moody, M. and Grocott, P. (1993) Let us extend our knowledge, assessment and management of fungating malignant wounds. *Professional Nurse*, **8**(9), 586–90.
Morris Docker, S. (1993) Effects of the European Community Directive on Lifting and Handling. *Professional Nurse*, **8**(10), 644–9.
National Back Pain Association/Royal College of Nursing (1993) *Mind Your Back: Patient Handling Guidelines*, NBPA/RCN, London.
Peate, I. (1993) Nurse administered oral hygiene in the hospitalized patient. *British Journal of Nursing*, **2**(9), 459–62.
Regnard, C. and Tempest, S. (1992) *A Guide to Symptom Relief in Advanced Cancer*, 3rd edn. Haigh and Hochland, Manchester.
Stone, C. (1993) Prescribed hydration in palliative care. *British Journal of Nursing*, **2**(7), 353–7.
Twycross, R.G. (1984) *A Time to Die*, CMF Publications, London.
Twycross, R.G. (1986) *The Dying Patient*, CMF Publications, London.

5 The problems of pain for the dying patient

WHAT IS PAIN?

The International Association for the Study of Pain defines pain as follows:

> Pain is an unpleasant sensory and emotional experience associated with actual or potential tissue damage, or described in terms of such damage. Pain is always subjective. Each individual learns the application of the word through experiences related to injury in early life. It is unquestionably a sensation in a part of the body but it is also unpleasant and therefore an emotional experience.

In caring for dying patients where pain is a prominent symptom, the majority will be in the terminal stage of cancer. To achieve successful pain relief, health care workers in the field must have a special understanding of pain and its effects on the sufferer. This section will therefore concentrate specifically on the management of pain due to malignant disease, but most will be applicable to patients dying from other causes and who are also in pain.

Pain is one of the commonest symptoms for cancer patients and often the most feared. Cancer patients often feel that pain is an inevitable part of their illness. The sense of hopelessness and the fear of impending death add to the total suffering of patients and exacerbate their pain. Reports show, however, that about two thirds of patients have pain and one third do not. The prevalence of pain increases as the disease progresses and varies depending on the primary site of the cancer.

Pain is a complex issue and unrelieved pain destroys quality of life. Pain is not, however, solely a reflection of tissue damage. The concept of 'total pain' recognizes the psychological, social and spiritual factors as well as the physical. Failure to consider all of these elements is likely to result in unsatisfactory management. Pain is therefore whatever the patient says it is and requires a systematic and sensitive approach to its management.

Chronic pain is disabling and distressing to the patient and their family. Individual and cultural variations exist. The associated uncertainty, fear and despair have negative effects on morale and exacerbate pain. Conversely explanation, reassurance rest and support help raise morale and increase pain threshold.

THE PAIN PATHWAYS

A number of nerve pathways, neurotransmitters and receptors have been identified as being involved in the perception of pain. The relationship between these pathways and the complexity of pain, however, remains unclear. Our current understanding of the mechanisms involved remains incomplete with models and theories going in and out of fashion. The description given below is a simple one; the network of connections within the pathways and between other pathways must be more complicated than that described to account for the observed complexity in the perception of pain.

Pain is perceived by free nerve endings in the tissues (**nociceptors**). Chemical mediators stimulate the nerve endings when tissue damage occurs and impulses are sent to the spinal cord. Bradykinin, prostaglandins, substance P, 5-hydroxytryptamine, noradrenaline and histamine are amongst the substances involved. The basis of the nerve impulse is electrochemical.

Pain impulses are transmitted to the central nervous system by two types of fibres called A δ fibres and C fibres. A δ fibres are myelinated, 2–5 μm in diameter and conduct at rates of 12–30 metres per second; they are thought to be responsible for distinct, sharp, well-defined and localized pain. C fibres are unmyelinated, 0.4–1.2 μm in diameter and conduct at rates of 0.5–2 metres per second; they are thought to give rise to diffuse, unpleasant, dull pain. The nerve fibres enter the spinal cord through its dorsal root in an area called the substantia gelatinosa (Fig. 5.1). This area is divided into six areas and contains a number of neurotransmitters.

It has been proposed that information entering the spinal cord, and the onward transmission of information to the higher centres of the brain, are regulated in the substantia gelatinosa. The 'gate theory' of Melzack and Wall in 1965 proposed a mechanism where nerve fibres from higher centres or at spinal cord level have an inhibitory or partial inhibitory effect on incoming information. When the inhibitory fibres are stimulated the 'gate' is closed and pain signals fail to reach consciousness.

After synapsing in the dorsal root the neurones cross the midline and ascend the spinal cord in the anterior and lateral columns as the spi-

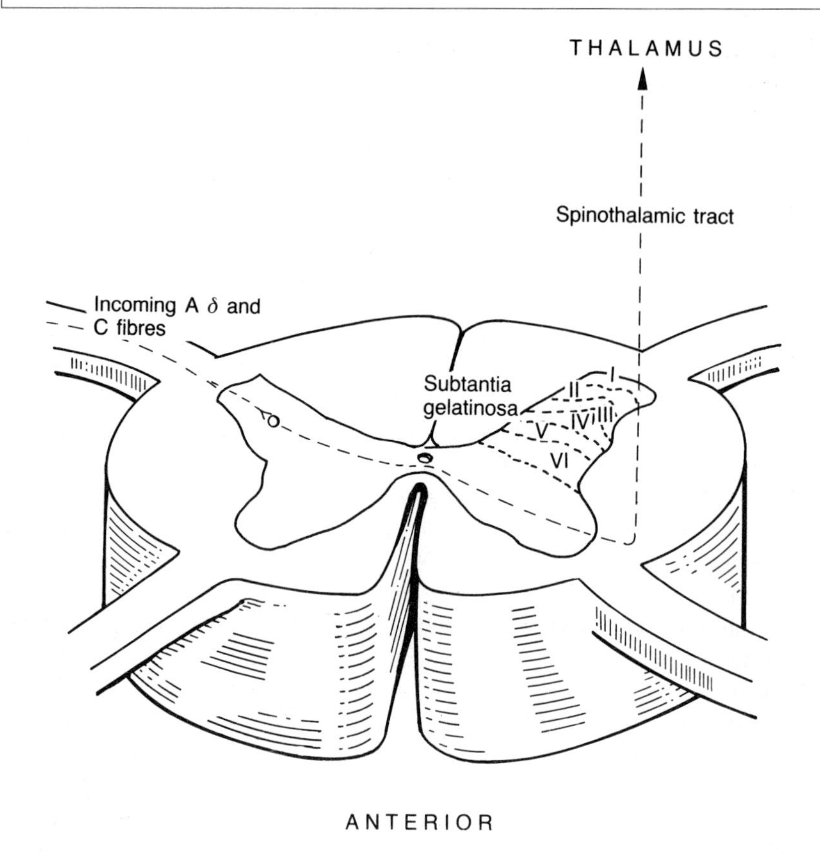

Figure 5.1 Cross-section through spinal cord to show incoming A δ and C fibres and substantia gelatinosa.

nothalamic tract to synapse in the thalamus. A δ fibres are thought to have a direct course to the thalamus and then on to the higher centres. C fibres, however, are thought to have connections with the reticular activating system of the brain. This area is concerned with mood and arousal.

The central nervous system produces its own natural analgesic substances. Endorphins and enkephalins, first isolated in 1975, work by binding to specific receptors in the body. Activation of these receptors inhibits the activity of the pain fibres and produces pain relief. Receptors initially found in the central nervous system have subsequently been found in the lung, iris and gut. There exist a family of receptors of which the principal subtypes have been designated μ, κ, δ and σ.

Most opioid analgesics used in cancer pain exert their effect by stimulation of the μ receptors. Stimulation of the δ and κ receptors is known to produce analgesia; however, the exact roles, particularly with κ receptors, is unclear. σ receptors may not be solely opioid receptors. The future development of more selective receptor agonists may produce better analgesic drugs.

ASSESSMENT OF PAIN

The effective management of pain requires a full understanding of the nature of pain as presented by the patient. Each patient perceives, describes and reacts to pain differently and assessment may be difficult. Physical, psychological, social and environmental factors all influence pain but the degree to which they do so must be explored.

Patients often have more than one pain and each pain may have a separate cause. Most pains are due to the cancer (Table 5.1). Some pains will be due to the treatments (e.g. surgery, chemotherapy or radiotherapy), some to debility (constipation, bedsores) and some to concurrent disorders unrelated to cancer. Each pain will require its own management plan based on the diagnosis.

The initial assessment is a baseline on which to plan management and monitor progress. It follows the normal medical model of history taking, physical examination and investigation (e.g. X-ray). Both the patient and the family should be involved as they have different perspectives to offer. Once the pains have been identified they will require individual assessment (Table 5.2). A number of methods have been used to allow the assessment to be objective, namely pain charts, visual analogue scales, pain diaries and questionnaires. Any analgesics used should be documented including doses and routes of administration, length of time taken, effectiveness and any adverse effects.

Following assessment a management plan must be agreed upon. The patient and their family should have the situation explained to them in language they will understand. Treatment options should be presented and the benefits and risks outlined. Realistic goals should be set so that

Table 5.1 Causes of cancer pain

Bone metastases
Nerve compression
Nerve infiltration
Nerve destruction
Soft tissue infiltration
Visceral pain
Lymphoedema
Raised intracranial pressure

Table 5.2 Individual assessment of pain

S	**S**ite
O	**O**rigin
C	**C**haracter
R	**R**adiation
A	**A**lleviating factors
T	**T**ime course
E	**E**xacerbating factors
S	**S**everity

the patient and family will know what to expect and what to do if the goals are not achieved. Analgesia should be given regularly and titrated to the individual's needs with the needs reassessed on a regular basis. Throughout the management empathy, understanding, explanation and ongoing support will have an analgesic effect in itself.

Bone pain

Bone is a metabolically active organ. It is constantly undergoing remodelling with a balance between bone resorption and new bone formation. Cancer cells attracted to the bone surface secrete products which interfere with these normal metabolic processes. If there is excess resorption lytic lesions result and if there is excess formation sclerotic lesions result.

Bone metastases are the most common cause of pain in cancer patients, accounting for almost half of all cancer pains. The spine, ribs and pelvis are frequently involved and the most common primary cancers are breast, lung, prostate, thyroid and kidney.

Pain may be described as dull or aching and is made worse by movement or direct pressure. The diagnosis is confirmed by X-ray or bone scan. There is no correlation between the size of the lesion and the amount of pain. The patient may present with a fracture as the first sign of disease.

Table 5.3 Treatment of bone pain

Non-steroidal anti-inflammatory drugs
Radiotherapy
Morphine
Internal fixation
Chemotherapy
Hormone therapy
Biphosphates
Steroids
Nerve block

The options for treatment of bone pain are outlined in Table 5.3. Bone pain is partially responsive to morphine and other treatments are usually also necessary.

Nerve pain

This may be caused by compression, infiltration or destruction of nerves. Management of nerve pain depends on the cause. Patients may present with a mixed picture which may complicate treatment.

Nerve compression as a result of malignancy usually presents as an aching, throbbing pain radiating along the course of the affected nerve. There may be an associated sensory loss and weakness. The resulting symptoms arise from a combination of the tumour and surrounding oedema.

Treatment is primarily with corticosteroids, as their anti-inflammatory effect relieves pressure by resolution of the tissue swelling and oedema. The remaining ache may be helped with morphine. If compression is associated with a bone metastasis or soft tissue tumour, radiotherapy is useful.

Infiltration or destruction of nerves leads to pain in an area of abnormal sensation – so-called neuropathic or deafferentation pain. This type of pain is distinguished from tissue damage in that it does not seem to involve the classic pain pathways. Neuropathic pain responds poorly, if at all, to morphine. In some cases neuropathic pain seems to depend upon the integrity of the sympathetic element of the autonomic nervous system.

Patients usually describe neuropathic pain as burning, stabbing or shooting. It is usually felt superficially in the area supplied by the nerve. It may be exacerbated by touch and the skin may feel warm. The pain is made worse by physical or emotional stress.

The choice of medication depends upon the presenting symptom(s). Antidepressants are helpful if there is a burning element to the pain. Anticonvulsants can be added if there is a shooting component. The membrane stabilizing drugs mexiletine and flecainide are useful second-line treatments. If the pain is maintained by the sympathetic nervous system a regional sympathetic block would be indicated. Transcutaneous nerve stimulation and acupuncture also have a role in the management of neuropathic pain.

Visceral pain

Results from the involvement of thoracic and/or abdominal viscera. Pain may result from distension or traction (liver capsule pain), obstruction (bowel, ureter) or irritation (bladder spasm, tenesmus). The effectiveness of morphine depends on the cause, but other treatments are often necessary.

Liver capsule pain occurs in about half the patients with liver metastases and is due to a stretching of the organ's capsule. Pain is usually in the right upper quadrant of the abdomen. It is helped by morphine. Other options include corticosteroids, radiotherapy, chemotherapy and a nerve block.

Colic is a feature of intestinal, renal and biliary obstruction. It does not respond well to morphine and in the case of biliary obstruction may be made worse. Hyoscine butylbromide (Buscopan) sublingually or subcutaneously is helpful. Surgery to alleviate the obstruction may be appropriate.

Bladder spasm causes intermittent suprapubic pain. It is helped by the anticholinergic oxybutynin hydrochloride. Other options include instillation of local anaesthetics into the bladder and a lumbar sympathetic nerve block. Tenesmus is an unpleasant sensation of wanting to open the bowels. It may be helped by morphine; alternatively radiotherapy, steroids (oral or rectal) and lumbar sympathetic nerve block may be considered.

Lymphoedema

This is the accumulation of lymph in the subcutaneous tissues. In cancer patients this is usually due to disease in the lymph nodes or blood vessels or to damage to lymph nodes or blood vessels following surgery or radiotherapy. The swelling may involve the limbs or trunk and is sometimes complicated by inflammation or infection of the skin.

Patients complain of tightness and heaviness with stretching of the skin. Although lymphoedema cannot be cured the symptoms can be controlled. The mainstay of treatment is physical (Table 5.4). Corticosteroids and diuretics may be used but they are of limited value.

Table 5.4 Management of lymphoedema

Exercises
Containment hosiery
Massage
Compression bandages
Intermittent pneumatic compression

Raised intracranial pressure

This may result from either primary or secondary tumours. The symptoms are due to a combination of tumour mass, reactive cerebral oedema and obstruction of the cerebrospinal fluid. About 10% of cancer patients present with brain metastases commonly from cancers originating in lung, breast and gastrointestinal tract.

The patient usually, but not invariably, complains of headache, the position of which does not always correlate with the site of disease. The headache, which is due to compression and distortion of the dura and blood vessels, is made worse by coughing or bending. The patient may feel drowsy and complain of nausea and vomiting. Examination may reveal swelling of the optic disc. Plain X-rays are rarely of value in making the diagnosis but computerized tomography and magnetic resonance imaging are more helpful.

Treatment is with high dose corticosteroids which will resolve the cerebral oedema. Radiotherapy is helpful in reducing tumour size and often carried out in combination with corticosteroid treatment. For patients with single lesions and no other sign of disease surgery may be appropriate.

ANALGESICS

Most cancer pain can be controlled with the use of oral analgesics and/or adjuvant drugs. An analgesic drug is one that relieves pain through either a central or peripheral effect (e.g. opioids, aspirin). Adjuvant drugs or co-analgesics are drugs used alongside analgesics in the control of pain but are not themselves analgesics (e.g. antidepressants).

A systematic approach to pain control is essential and includes setting realistic objectives, administering regular medication and regular review and reassessment. In 1986 the World Health Organization published simple guidelines on the use of drugs for cancer pain based on the clinical experience of a number of international units. The guidelines, presented in the form of an 'analgesic ladder' (Fig. 5.2), recommend that mild pain is treated with a non-opioid analgesic with or without adjuvant medication. If the pain increases a weak opioid should be introduced. If the pain becomes severe a strong opioid should be substituted for the weak opioid.

Aspirin, codeine and morphine are examples of the drugs used at the three stages of the ladder. The dose of each drug is maximized at the lower steps before reaching morphine which has no maximum dose. Alternatives to the three analgesics may be used depending on circumstances (Table 5.5). Medication is usually administered orally but other

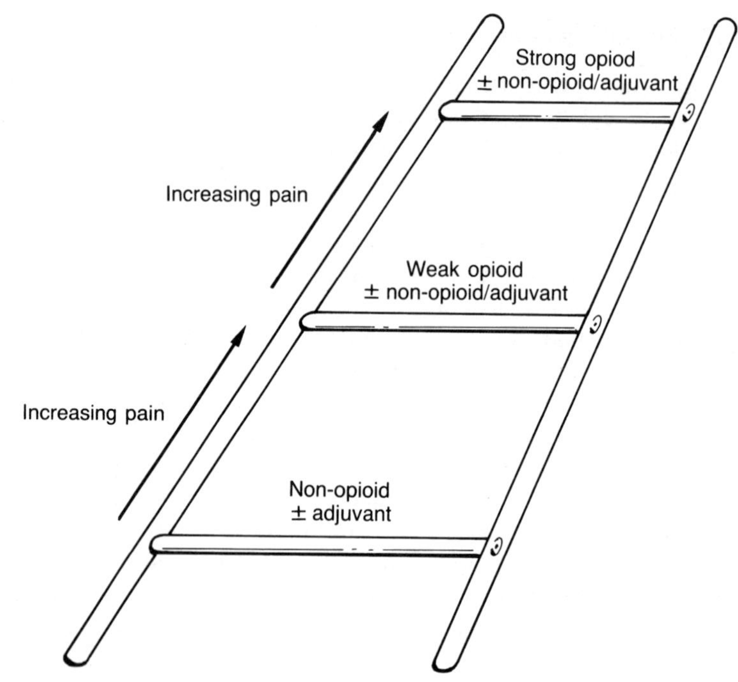

Figure 5.2 The World Health Organization's analgesic ladder.

Table 5.5 Analgesics used in the analgesic ladder

NSAIDS	WEAK OPIOIDS	STRONG OPIOIDS
Aspirin	Codeine	Morphine
Ibuprofen	Dihydrocodeine	Diamorphine
Naproxen	Dextropropoxyphene	Oxycodone
Indomethacin		Dextromoramide
		Phenazocine
		Methadone
		Pentazocine
		Buprenorphine

routes may be used including sublingual, rectal, subcutaneous, transdermal and spinal.

Non-steroidal anti-inflammatory drugs (NSAIDs)

NSAIDs are derived from a number of chemical substances. The main groups are salicylic acid, arylalcanoic acid, anthrananilic acid, pyrazolone, indole and indene compounds. In regular full dosage NSAIDs have an analgesic and anti-inflammatory effect. The difference in anti-inflammatory activity between the different NSAIDs is small but there is variation in their analgesic effect. About 60% of patients respond to any NSAID, another 20% respond on changing the NSAID and 20% have a poor response. The incidence and type of side effect vary with NSAIDs. The main side effects include indigestion, gastrointestinal haemorrhage, nausea and fluid retention.

Aspirin

Derived from salicyclic acid, aspirin was first marketed in 1899. It is available in over-the-counter preparations. Aspirin has antipyretic, anti-inflammatory and analgesic effects. It exerts its action by blocking the synthesis of prostaglandins, substances produced as a result of tissue damage and thought to directly stimulate free nerve endings resulting in pain. It may also have a central analgesic action. Aspirin is absorbed mainly from the stomach.

The dose used is between 600 mg and 1000 mg 4-hourly. Side effects may occur at any dose and it is important to ascertain if any predisposing factors exist. A number of preparations exist, including enteric coating, which may be better tolerated.

There are numerous other NSAIDs available but the incidence of side effects usually increases with the potency of the preparation. It is useful to become familiar with a small number of preparations so that they may be used with confidence. Three commonly used NSAIDs are ibuprofen, naproxen and indomethacin. **Ibuprofen** is a mild NSAID; the daily dose is 1.2–2.8 g. **Naproxen** is a medium strength NSAID; the daily dose is 0.5–1 g. **Indomethacin** is a strong NSAID; the daily dose is 50–200 mg. All three preparations are given in divided doses.

Paracetamol is not an NSAID but is useful for mild pain. It is an anti-prostaglandin and has analgesic and antipyretic properties but no anti-inflammatory properties. It has fewer gastrointestinal side effects than NSAIDs and may therefore be better tolerated. The usual dose is 0.5–1 g 6-hourly. It is also available in combination with aspirin as benorylate (usual dose 5–10 ml twice daily) which is said to have fewer side effects than aspirin alone.

Opioid analgesics

This is a group of naturally occurring and synthetic substances. Opium itself is derived from dried juice of the seed capsule of *Papaver somniferum*, a poppy indigenous to Asia. Accounts of its use exist in Egyptian, Greek and Roman cultures when it was used to induce sleep and

Table 5.6 Approximate daily morphine equivalent of opioids

Opioid	Route	Conversion*
Morphine	Oral	1
Morphine	Subcutaneous	2
Codeine	Oral	0.08
Dihydrocodeine	Oral	0.1
Dextropropoxyphene	Oral	0.16
Diamorphine	Oral	1.5
Diamorphine	Subcutaneous	3
Oxycodone	Rectal	1
Dextromoramide	Oral	2
Phenazocine	Oral/sublingual	5
Methadone	Oral	3.5
Buprenorphine	Sublingual	70

*Multiply daily dose of opiate by conversion factor

euphoria. The main constituents of the poppy seed are morphine, codeine, noscapine, papavarine and thebaine. The main actions of opium are due to its morphine content.

Opioids have both a stimulant and depressant effect on the central nervous system. The difference between preparations is due to differences in receptor binding. In practice the decision to use a particular preparation is based on the presence (or absence) of a maximum dose, oral efficacy, speed of action, duration of action and unwanted side effects. The equivalent doses of opioids compared to morphine are shown in Table 5.6.

Codeine is methylmorphine. Ten percent of codeine is metabolized to morphine, so it is therefore less effective than morphine as an analgesic. It is indicated in the treatment of mild to moderate pain. It is also helpful in treating cough and as an antidiarrhoeal agent.

Codeine exists in strengths of 15 mg, 30 mg and 60 mg. The routine dose is between 30–60 mg 4–6-hourly. If pain is not relieved at the maximum dose morphine should be commenced. Codeine is also available in combination with non-opioids, aspirin and paracetamol.

Dihydrocodeine is a semisynthetic analogue of codeine with a similar potency. The usual dose is 30–60 mg 4–6-hourly. A slow release preparation exists which is given 12-hourly and may aid compliance. **Dextropropoxyphene** is a synthetic derivative of methadone. Given alone it is a mild analgesic and less potent than codeine. It is commonly given in combination with paracetamol as coproxamol (dextropropoxyphene 32.5 mg and paracetamol 325 mg).

Table 5.7 Side effects of morphine

Constipation	Nausea and vomiting
Drowsiness	Confusion
Hallucinations	Pupillary constriction
Euphoria and relaxation	Myoclonic jerks
Respiratory depression	Tolerance
Dependence	Pruritus

Morphine is the opioid of choice for the oral treatment of severe cancer pain. It is, however, as important to know when not to use morphine as when to use it. Most but not all cancer pains respond well to morphine. Some pains respond partially (bone metastases), some pains do not respond (nerve destruction) and some may be made worse (constipation).

When taken orally morphine is absorbed from the small intestine. It is metabolized principally in the liver to form two main metabolites, morphine-3-glucuronide (M3G) and morphine-6-glucuronide (M6G). M6G stimulates the μ receptors and accounts for the analgesic action of morphine. M3G has no significant analgesic effect and in some situations may antagonize the analgesic effects of morphine.

Morphine causes side effects both inside and outside the central nervous system (Table 5.7), which are not dose related. Some side effects are transitory (nausea and vomiting) whilst others may be permanent (constipation). Respiratory depression, tolerance and dependence are not clinically a problem in cancer patients if the dose of morphine is titrated to the pain.

There is no 'standard dose' of morphine; the single most important factor in determining the dose is the patient's pain. The usual starting dose is 10 mg 4-hourly. Increments in response to pain are usually of the order of 25–50% and are made to prevent the pain returning before the next dose of medication is due.

Morphine is available as solution, tablet or suppository with a 4-hour duration of action. Alternatively slow release tablets or dissolvable granules with a 12-hourly duration of action are available.

Diamorphine (heroin) is a semisynthetic substance first made from morphine in 1874 at St Mary's Hospital in London and first introduced in 1898. In the body it is metabolized first to morphine. Its advantage over morphine is in parenteral administration because of its greater solubility. It is commonly used in syringe drivers. Like morphine it has no maximum dose.

Oxycodone is a synthetic derivative of morphine. It is obtained by special order and is available as a suppository at a dose of 30 mg. The advantage of oxycodone over morphine suppositories is its 8-hourly action and hence less frequent administration.

Dextromoramide may be less sedating and is shorter acting than morphine. It is helpful for breakthrough pain and for painful procedures. The oral dose is 5–20 mg. It is also available as a suppository.

Phenazocine is a synthetic analgesic which is effective both orally and sublingually. It acts rapidly and has a longer action than morphine. It is helpful for patients having troublesome side effects from morphine. The usual dose is 5–20 mg.

Methadone is a synthetic drug with effects similar to morphine but with a longer period of action. The usual dose is 5–10 mg given twice daily to avoid accumulation.

Pentazocine is a synthetic derivative of phenazocine. It is a strong analgesic but also has antagonist properties. The dose is 25–100 mg 3–4-hourly.

Buprenorphine has both agonist and antagonist properties. Its duration of action is approximately 6–8 hours. It does not have an upper dose and is available in 0.2 mg and 0.4 mg preparations which are taken sublingually.

Co-analgesic drugs

Tricyclic antidepressants

This group of drugs is helpful in the management of neuropathic pain, particularly if associated with unpleasant sensory changes. The mode of action is not completely understood. Monoamine neurotransmitters in the brain are known to increase and these may stimulate descending pain inhibitory pathways.

Amitriptyline 25 mg at night increasing to 100 mg at night normally results in improvement of pain within a week. This analgesic effect is separate from its antidepressant effect which takes longer. Lofepramine 35–70 mg at night and dothiepin 75 mg at night are alternatives.

Anticonvulsants

These drugs are indicated in the management of neuropathic pain, particularly if there is a stabbing component. The mechanism of action is thought to be through its membrane stabilizing properties.

Carbamezepine 100 mg at night increasing to 400 mg 12-hourly or alternatively sodium valproate 500 mg at night increasing to 1 g are useful. An improvement is noted within a week.

Corticosteroids

This group of drugs has a wide application in cancer patients. They help produce analgesia by reducing oedema and inflammation surrounding tumour, thereby relieving pressure on surrounding tissue. They are helpful in nerve compression, raised intracranial pressure, spinal cord compression and organ infiltration. At low doses they increase general well-being and therefore can increase pain threshold.

Dexamethasone and prednisolone are both useful. Dexamethasone is usually preferred as it is more potent, so fewer tablets are required, and there is less fluid retention. The dose depends on the problem: 2–4 mg is helpful for appetite, 8–12 mg is helpful in nerve compression and organ infiltration, 16–24 mg is used in raised intracranial pressure and as much as 96 mg has been used in spinal cord compression.

Hormone therapy

In some cancers hormone treatment will modify the pathological process and thus relieve pain. The effect is thought to be due to interaction with specific receptors on tumours. Two examples where hormones are commonly used are carcinoma of the breast and prostate.

About half the patients with breast cancer benefit from hormonal therapy. Tamoxifen, an oestrogen antagonist, is the commonest preparation. The daily dose is 20–40 mg. Aminoglutethamide 250 mg daily is an alternative choice.

A lowering of plasma male hormone levels will help the majority of patients with carcinoma of the prostate. Cyproterone acetate is an anti-androgen and is useful first-line therapy. The usual dose is 100 mg three times daily. Goserelin, a monthly depot injection, is also helpful.

Antibiotics

Cancer patients have an increased susceptibility to infections. The cancer itself, the treatment (e.g. chemotherapy) and the associated debility make bacterial, fungal and viral infections common. Most infections cause pain and discomfort which will resolve with treatment of the underlying cause.

Whenever possible specimens should be sent for microbiological analysis: microscopy, culture and sensitivity. Prescribing is usually limited to oral preparations. The choice of antibiotic will depend on the patient, the causative organism (if known) and local prescribing policies.

Antispasmodics

Cancer patients are often troubled by colic resulting from tumour obstruction. A common problem is the colic resulting from bowel obstruction.

Intestinal colic may be reduced by loperamide 2–4 mg four times daily.

Alternatively hyoscine hydrobromide given sublingually at a dose of 0.3 mg three times daily or as a subcutaneous infusion may be used.

Muscle relaxants

This group of drugs is helpful in the management of muscle spasm. This may be following limb paralysis, immobility or sometimes associated with bone lesions.

Diazepam 5–10 mg daily in divided doses or baclofen 5–10 mg three times daily is useful.

Co-analgesic therapies

Approximately 10% of patients have pain that is difficult to control with oral medication. There are instances, therefore, when the input of specialities outside the hospice or community setting is appropriate. Radiotherapists, oncologists, anaesthetists and surgeons are part of the multidisciplinary team available to contribute to the patient's management. This management will usually take place in a hospital.

The aims of any treatment must be clear at the outset and the patient involved in the decisions. Pain relief may be obtained by modifying the tumour growth with radiotherapy and chemotherapy and interrupting nerve pathways either surgically or chemically. These processes, however, are not without side effects in terms of physical toxicity and psychosocial morbidity. The decision for appropriate management may be difficult.

Radiotherapy

Over 50% of cancer patients receive radiotherapy; in one third of patients the treatment is palliative. Radiotherapy acts by breaking down cellular DNA. The body then removes the damaged cells. As normal cells are able to repair their damaged DNA more effectively than tumour cells, the cancer is selectively targeted.

Careful planning prior to treatment is essential. The effectiveness of treatment has been aided by advances in imaging techniques (e.g. computerized tomography and magnetic resonance imaging) allowing precise mapping of tumours and by advances in the quality and penetrating power of radiotherapy equipment. Also to be considered prior to treatment are the radiosensitivity of the tumour and the amount of previous radiotherapy, if any, to the area.

Radiotherapy may be considered in a number of painful conditions (Table 5.8). The aim of treatment is to relieve pain quickly with the lowest possible dose and with the fewest possible treatments, as treatment is not without side effects. These include nausea, vomiting, diarrhoea,

Table 5.8 Role of radiotherapy in pain

Bone metastases
Nerve entrapment
Fungating wound
Dysphagia
Pelvic pain due to tumour
Chest pain due to tumour
Raised intracranial pressure
Venous obstruction
Lymphatic obstruction
Spinal cord compression

oesophagitis, alopecia, mucositis and dry mouth. The incidence and type of side effects depend on the site and dose of irradiation.

Chemotherapy

Cytotoxic drugs are those that cause direct damage to cells and are most useful against actively dividing cells. Cytotoxics fall into a number of classes including alkylating drugs, cytotoxic antibiotics, antimetabolites, vinca alkaloids and etoposide. Each class has its own characteristic anti-tumour activity, sites of action and toxic effects. Cytotoxics may be used either singly or in combination. Not all tumours respond to chemotherapy; the relief of pain is therefore more likely in those tumours that do (Table 5.9).

Side effects are common and include nausea, vomiting, mucositis, marrow suppression, bleeding, infections and alopecia. It is important to determine the objectives and the treatment plan at the outset and review and revise treatment based on the progress, including troublesome side effects.

Table 5.9 Cancers in which chemotherapy is useful

Breast (advanced)	Head and neck
Lung	Kidney
Alimentary tract	Urinary bladder
Ovarian	Brain
Endometrium	Melanoma
Cervix	Soft tissue sarcoma
Low grade non-Hodgkin's lymphoma	

Table 5.10 Principal nerve blocks for cancer pain

Intercostal
Paravertebral
Coeliac plexus
Sacral
Brachial plexus
Intrathecal
Epidural

Anaesthetic techniques

Anaesthetists will carry out simple techniques in hospices, but most procedures usually require hospital facilities. If based in pain clinics, four modes of treatment are offered: drugs, nerve blocks, nerve stimulation (e.g. acupuncture, transcutaneous nerve stimulation, implanted stimulators) and psychological techniques.

Several nerve blocks are used to complement oral medication in the control of cancer pain (Table 5.10). Nerve blocks are particularly helpful when pain is controlled at rest but not on movement or when localized pain breaks through otherwise well controlled pain.

In principle, pain pathways are interrupted so that messages do not reach the higher centres and pain is not perceived. A number of procedures may be used including local anaesthetic agents (bupivacaine), neurolytic agents (phenol, alcohol, glycerol) and physical agents (cryoanalgesia, radiofrequency). Drugs may be administered spinally through either a percutaneous catheter or a fully implanted system. Morphine and other drugs injected epidurally and intrathecally have been shown to relieve pain.

Table 5.11 Surgical procedures in cancer patients

Relief of intestinal obstruction
Relief of urinary obstruction
Decompression of spinal cord
Internal fixation of pathological fracture
Prophylactic internal fixation of bone metastases
Cordotomy
Pituitary ablation
Oophorectomy
Orchidectomy
Resection of solitary metastasis
Resection of brain tumour
Debridement of necrotic wound
Incision and drainage of abscess

Surgery

There are a number of situations where surgical intervention would be appropriate for the patient with cancer related pain (Table 5.11). Patients may also present with pain from concurrent disorders normally requiring surgical management (e.g. appendicitis, perforated viscus).

Patients where surgery is considered are usually stable (unless the operation is carried out as an emergency), their disease not widespread and they are agreeable to this option. Surgery is inappropriate in cases where the patient is too unwell and there is widespread disease.

SUMMARY

- The nature of pain is complex.
- Our understanding of the pain pathways is incomplete.
- A complete assessment of the pain is essential.
- Both the patient and the family should participate in the assessment of pain.
- Diagnose the cause and then treat.
- Pain can usually be controlled with oral analgesics.
- Management should be systematic.
- Management is most effective in a multidisciplinary setting.
- The WHO analgesic ladder provides a basis for treating cancer pain.
- Review and reassess beneficial effects and side effects of treatment.

NURSING MANAGEMENT OF THE PATIENT WITH PAIN

The nurse has a powerful and responsible position with regard to pain. She is often the key person to resolve whether the patient's pain gets better or worse, since nurses provide a continuous service to patients and are thus in a position to convey to the doctor an accurate picture of the pattern of pain. As the nurse spends more time with the patient than any other team member, she is often the sole person able to evaluate the efficacy of the treatment and monitor any changes in the type or location of pain. This entails developing skills of observation in which all aspects of the symptoms are perceived and understood.

Attitudes and communications

If nurses are to help patients they must accept that pain is a subjective experience. Any sensing by patients that the reality and degree of their pain are doubted will have a detrimental effect. Depression will occur, if not already present, and this is likely to intensify the pain, since tension and depression are interrelated. A guiding principle should be 'Pain is whatever the experiencing person says it is' (McCaffery, 1983). This is fundamental to nursing the patient effectively and is linked with the conviction that pain is affected by the emotions that may be experienced by the dying patient, notably fear. Indeed, fear of pain that will become increasingly intolerable is not uncommonly the most prominent feature in many people's expectation of dying. When the dying patient is actually suffering from unrelieved and severe pain, this becomes a vicious circle with fear exacerbating the pain.

In assessing the needs of a dying patient, the ability to recognize cues regarding pain experience is crucial. There must be time to listen to the patient's description of that pain, to watch for non-verbal signs, for example, facial expression, posture and sounds such as moaning, rapid breathing or sighing.

Sometimes the nurse will experience inward distress at witnessing pain not yet adequately relieved in a dying person. In such a difficult situation where, despite efforts by the caring team, the problem is not yet resolved, there may even be a temptation for the carer to avoid the patient because of these painful emotions.

Nurses also have their own individual personalities and bring to their work learnt attitudes to pain and illness behaviour (Latham, 1987). It is important to recognize this and the trained nurse could, with benefit, discuss the matter with the student nurse when there is a problem.

The nurse needs to develop a positive attitude towards the availability of resources to control pain. These include not only the use of drugs and various therapies the doctor will initiate and the nurse will be responsible for maintaining, but also a number of other means of relieving pain the nurse can operate alone.

It has been mentioned that individuals all have their own pain thresholds, so that one person will not be able to tolerate easily a level of pain or discomfort that another will find hardly worth mentioning. This difference is influenced by the patient's unique personal history, including cultural factors (Sofaer, 1984). Where it is proving difficult to assess pain in a dying patient, it may be useful for the nurse to use a pain chart such as those developed by Raiman (1981). A pain assessment chart provides a systematic approach to enable nurses to assess and document the patient's pain effectively. It is essential to carry out regular pain assessment as the patient's symptoms may change frequently, especially in the final stages of disease.

Some methods of pain relief

It must be accepted that the nature of pain, its causes and relief are not fully understood; therefore it is necessary to work **with** the patient to alleviate his or her pain. New information is constantly unfolding in this field and can enhance understanding of how to manage individual pain control. For instance, it is now recognized that the use of placebos will relieve actual physical pain and that this does not mean that the patient is a malingerer.

Being with the patient

Simply staying with patients can contribute to pain relief. This is because anxiety and other distressing emotions may be lessened by the patient's feeling of confidence that they are not left alone, especially with anticipatory fears that the pain will return.

It also gives patients the opportunity to gain relief from some of the mental pain that may be afflicting them and they may choose to unburden themselves to the nurse who is giving their company. Thoughts of impending loss of everything that life holds for them, terror at the idea of death coming in a violent manner or a sense of frustration at what seems in retrospect a life containing little tangible achievement call for compassionate and unhurried listening. 'Physical and mental suffering are closely interwoven and a division into bodily and mental pain is an artificial one' (Lamerton, 1980). The introduction in many units of primary and team nursing means the nurse is able to spend more time with a smaller group of patients. If the nurse can build up a trusting relationship this can reduce the patient's anxiety and thereby reduce their pain.

Achieving comfort of position

The patient may find it difficult to achieve a comfortable position in bed or chair, due to emaciation and thus pressure on bony prominences. Or oedema may be present, causing painful tension of swollen limbs or abdomen. The presence of pressure sores will add to the problem. In patients with cancer, the presence of bony secondary deposits calls for very careful handling by the nurse both to avoid causing pain and also because of the risk of pathological fractures.

Patients themselves and their relatives may have found the best way of sitting or lying to avoid pain and the most comfortable arrangement of pillows and the nurse should accept their advice. A variety of positions may be adopted and plenty of pillows should be available; the large triangular pillow is often valued. Patients with neck lesions need special attention; sometimes a cervical collar is helpful or small neck pillows. Other aids to comfort in bed or sitting in a chair that are commonly used in nursing for many types of patient can all be of value to the dying patient in helping to relieve pain.

The patient with spinal metastases or spinal cord lesion will need particular attention. A firm-based bed is essential, as is careful positioning of limbs to prevent contractures. Some form of paralysis may be present and therefore all these points regarding position are of great importance. If the paralysis is of recent occurrence the patient will probably be anxious and frustrated by loss of function and need a sympathetic and positive approach from their carers. The help of a physiotherapist will be an asset to advise on suitable exercises and aids to support the paralysed limb. These include ripple beds, sheepskins to sit on or place under heels, and footstools.

Dealing with painful skin and mucous membranes

Since all systems of the body are linked together, the dying patient will have a number of physical discomforts to contend with, some of which may cause severe pain and not be directly caused by the main disease. The skin is a potent guide to the state of an individual's health and inevitably is at risk in the deteriorating dying body. Pressure sores may arise despite care or gravitational ulcers in the patient with cardiovascular disease. Preventive measures having failed, nursing care must be planned to minimize the pain and further breakdown of the skin and underlying tissue. If pressure sores or other skin lesions are present it is often the nurse's responsibility to decide which type of dressing will be used. This needs to be as comfortable as possible – both whilst in place and also during dressing changes. In the case of extensive or painful wounds, it may be necessary to give extra analgesia prior to changing the dressing. This will require judicious topical medication and relief of pressure on the area.

A painful mouth is very common and should always be anticipated in the dying patient by frequent topical care, using any special medication prescribed by the doctor. Severe ulceration with haemorrhage may occur, particularly in patients with leukaemia or end-stage renal failure, and is very painful. Dryness of the mouth adds to the discomfort and the nurse should use all measures to relieve this, realizing that the patient may not be able to draw attention to the problem (Chapter 4).

The presence of haemorrhoids is another condition that can cause much pain and misery to the dying patient, exacerbated if the patient tries to pass hard stools. Here, prevention of constipation is a serious responsibility on the nurse's part to avoid this largely unnecessary pain. If haemorrhoids, or anal fissure, are present, local application of suitable ointment or analgesic rectal suppositories should be used.

In women, the vulva may be a site for tenderness and pain if, for instance, a malignant lesion is present. A rectovaginal fistula will also result in an inflamed mucosa and be very painful because of the excretions passing over it. The pain is further compounded in the conscious patient by embarrassment and anxiety because of the site involved and the unpleasant smell that is often present. Here, the tact and gentleness of the nurse is all-important. Local treatment to soothe the inflammation and to maintain hygiene is required and care that the level of analgesic drugs the patient is receiving is appropriate to control the pain.

The bladder mucosa may become inflamed; cystitis is quite a common and very painful condition. Antibiotic therapy is usually prescribed unless the patient is near death. The nurse should also take the usual steps of seeing that the patient is taking as much fluid as possible and handle an indwelling catheter with scrupulous care to avoid further infection.

The patient may have an open wound that is extensive and painful. Malignant skin lesions, such as fungating carcinoma of breast, are unpleasant both for the patient and the nurse. Secondary infection is likely and an offensive odour. This is another example of pain with both a physical and mental component, needing analgesic drugs to control it, plus local dressings and some means of suppressing the odour such as an aerosol spray used in the room.

Headache

Like anyone else, a dying patient may suffer from an occasional headache which clears up quickly following administration of a mild analgesic such as aspirin.

Headaches may, however, have a grave cause, such as a brain tumour, or occur in end-stage renal failure. Here the headaches will be intense, prolonged and occur at frequent intervals. The pressure building up within the skull is due to excess cerebrospinal fluid and, in the case of a tumour, actual increase in size of the space-occupying lesion.

Temporary relief can often be obtained by giving large doses of steroid drugs which will reduce oedema in and around the tumour and thus the intracranial pressure. Unfortunately, a decision eventually has to be made as to how long this palliative treatment should continue.

Whether the headache is from a benign or malignant cause, the nurse can help to relieve the pain by using such time-honoured simple remedies as cold compresses to the forehead, shading the patient's eyes from bright lights and providing a quiet atmosphere.

Use of relaxation and distraction techniques

Relaxation can be defined as a state of freedom from both anxiety and skeletal muscle tension. Dying patients with pain are likely to be anxious and tense, which lowers their pain threshold. Simple techniques, such as getting patients into as comfortable a position as possible and instructing them to close their eyes and breathe rhythmically and deeply, can be used by the nurse. Sometimes soft, slow music may help and act as a distraction from the pain.

Distraction as a non-invasive pain relief method is a kind of sensory shielding, a protecting of oneself from the pain sensation by focusing on and increasing the clarity of sensations unrelated to pain (McCaffery, 1983). Nurses who wish to try this method need to know their patients well enough to judge what distraction would be most likely to help. For instance, if a patient is very keen on sporting events, the topic could be introduced and discussed for a brief period. Music has already been mentioned and the use of visual images such as showing patients a series of pictures likely to interest them is another example.

This whole field of non-invasive pain relief methods is a complex one and is arousing a good deal of interest for patients with chronic pain, including those in a terminal stage of illness. Cutaneous stimulation is another method that includes some ancient techniques, such as use of heat and cold applications to the body, massage and counterirritants and transcutaneous electric nerve stimulation. A further step, where the skin is actually penetrated, is acupuncture.

Some of these ideas may be used with benefit to the dying patient by the nurse and doctor working together or singly according to the degree of sophistication favoured. Special training is needed before using certain relaxation and distraction techniques and details of these are beyond the scope of this book.

Administration of drugs for control of pain

Since this is the main way of controlling physical pain, it is considered fitting to end this section by emphasizing again the crucial role of the nurse in the matter. The basic principles of safe administration of drugs are, of course, as important here as in any situation, especially as most of the drugs used will be opiates, i.e. controlled drugs. The nurse is often responsible for deciding how much medication to give and also whether extra analgesia is required between drug rounds. In this case it is often the nurse who decides what type of prescribed analgesia is appropriate for the patient's pain and by which route it should be given. The nurse's knowledge and education play an important part in pain control. For example, if the nurse does not understand the use of or has a fear of opiate addiction, the patient may not be offered adequate analgesia.

There are other aspects that need special mention:

1. Oral medication is used as much possible and the dying patient often needs help with this towards the end, when weakness is increasing and muscle coordination is difficult. An unhurried approach is essential.
2. Close monitoring of the effects of the drug will mainly fall on the

nurse. If the pain is unrelieved or has reappeared before the next dose is due, this must be reported as soon as possible to the doctor so that action can be taken to improve control of the pain. It is important that the nurse checks the effect of the drug about half an hour after it has been administered and then at least half an hour before the next dose is due.

3. When death is near, it should be remembered that if opiates have been given regularly to control pain, they must continue to be given even if the patient becomes semicomatose. If this principle is not followed and an opiate is suddenly discontinued, there may be withdrawal reactions and the patient may experience pain even though unable to communicate verbally. Drugs that hitherto have been taken orally will now have to be administered by suppositories or injection. The dose of the drug will continue to need careful assessment by the nurse and the doctor. Sometimes the amount may be reduced but occasionally there may be evidence of increasing pain requiring larger doses of opiates.
4. The use of the syringe driver

> 'A syringe driver must not be seen only as a means of prescribing drugs in the last few hours or days of life. It is a useful method of administering drugs when the oral route is, for various reasons not practical'. (T.F. Benton) 1991

Indications for use

- Impaired swallowing or intestinal absorption
- Persistent nausea and vomiting
- Extreme weakness
- Restlessness
- Pain poorly controlled by oral medication.

Advantages

- The patient is disturbed less frequently
- Fear, anxiety and the discomfort often caused by regular injections is avoided.

The Graseby Medical model MS 16a is commonly used, and consists of a light, portable, battery operated pump, which carries a syringe. The syringe is attached to a 'butterfly' needle which is inserted subcutaneously. Suitable sites include the chest and abdominal wall, thigh and upper arm.

Medication is given over 24 hours at a steady rate ensuring constant plasma concentration levels. Excellent symptom control can be achieved, often with reduced total drug dosage.

Before the syringe driver is set up, explanation must be given to the patient and relatives, and its use accepted.

Ambulant patients may maintain independence with the syringe driver being carried in a pouch worn around the waist or over the shoulder.

General care

- The needle site should be protected with a transparent dressing.
- The syringe should be protected from light.
- The needle site should be observed regularly for skin reaction. The site should be changed if this occurs.
- The insertion site is usually changed after 48 hours.
- Not all drugs can be safely mixed.

Examples

- METOCLOPRAMIDE, METHOTRIMEPRAZINE and HYOSCINE can all be mixed safely with Diamorphine.
- CYCLIZINE and HALOPERIDOL may both cause precipitation when mixed with DIAMORPHINE.

Patients and their relatives need to be assured that putting up with the pain is contrary to the goal being aimed for and that there is no question of the patient being considered cowardly or ungrateful if they give an accurate picture of inadequate relief. The qualified nurse also has a responsibility to educate their junior colleagues, e.g. student nurses, in the proper approach to pain control. Paying lip service to the principles is insufficient; attitudes are more often 'caught not taught'.

Nurses who act compassionately and intelligently with their medical colleagues in striving to reach the ideal situation of complete pain control render a considerable service to their dying patients.

REFERENCES

Lamerton, R. (1980) *Care of the Dying*, Pelican, Harmondsworth.

Latham, J. (1987) *Pain Control*, Lisa Sainsbury Foundation series, Austen Cornish, London.

McCaffery, M. (1983) *Nursing the Patient in Pain*, Harper and Row, London.

Raiman, J. (1981) Responding to pain. *Nursing*, **1**(31), 1362–5.

Sofaer, B. (1984) *Pain: A Handbook for Nurses*, Harper and Row, London.

FURTHER READING

Hayward, J. (1981) *Information – A Prescription against Pain*, Royal College of Nursing, London.

Hockey, L. (1981) *Recent Advances in Nursing 1: Current Issues in Nursing*, Churchill Livingstone, Edinburgh.

Kaye, P. (1992) *A–Z of Hospice and Palliative Medicine*, EPL Publications, Northampton.
Regnard, C.F.B. and Tempest, S. (1992) *A Guide to Symptom Relief in Advanced Cancer*, 3rd edn, Haigh and Hochland, Manchester.
Saunders, C. and Sykes, N. (eds) (1993) *The Management of Terminal Malignant Illness*, 3rd edn, Edward Arnold, London.
Twycross, R.G. and Lack, S.A. (1990) *Therapeutics in Terminal Care*, 2nd edn, Churchill Livingstone, London.
Watt-Watson, J.H. and Donovan, M.I. (1992) *Pain Management – Nursing Perspective*, Mosby Year Book, St Louis.
World Health Organization (1990) *Cancer Pain Relief and Palliative Care*, Report of a WHO Expert Committee, Technical Report Series 804, WHO, Geneva.

USE OF SYRINGE DRIVERS

REFERENCE

Doyle, D. and Benton, T.F., Palliative Medicine, Pain and Symptom Control, Edinburgh, (revised edition) 1991, St Columbas's Hospice,
quoted in; Helpful Essential Links to Palliative Care. University of Dundee and Cancer Relief Macmillan, 1992, page 86.

USEFUL READING

Regnard, C. and Tempest, S., *A Guide to Symptom Relief in Advanced Cancer*, 3rd edition, 1992, Haugh and Hochland Ltd, Manchester.
Pritchard, S., Evaluating Syringe Drivers, *Nursing Times*, 24th April, Vol. 87, No. 17, 1991, page 38–39.
Oliver, D., Syringe Drivers in the Community (Prescribing for the 90's), *The Practitioner*, January 1991, Vol. 235, page 78–80.
Helpful Essential Links to Palliative Care, University of Dundee and Cancer Relief Macmillan, 1992.

USEFUL ADDRESS

Graseby Medical Ltd,
Colonial Way
Watford
Hertfordshire
WD2 4LG
England

6 The last hours of life

Robert Twycross in his book *The Dying Patient* writes 'Death is probably the loneliest experience any of us will face' (Twycross, 1975).

As nurses care for patients during their last hours, they must remember that they are still unique individuals who have had control of their lives, probably for many years. They have made decisions, been consulted, communicated with many and loved and been loved.

Now as death comes, the despair and resentment which may have been present earlier and the increasing helplessness can add up to total isolation and become 'that loneliest experience'.

There may also be fears – fears of dying in pain, of losing all bodily control, of loss of dignity and of dying alone – the process of dying. It is perhaps worth considering, when trying to recognize these fears, whether it is possible to distinguish between the fear of death and the fear of dying.

Canon David Watson (cited in Twycross, 1984) in a BBC radio interview in April 1983 some time before his death from cancer, speaking as a committed Christian, acknowledged his fear of dying but had no fear of death. One of the compilers of this chapter vividly remembers the lasting impact this statement made on her.

Nurses and all other staff involved must strive to ensure that the patient does feel they matter and are of value and that they are still being consulted about their care. In meeting their needs, which may be mainly the relief of symptoms, it is important to ensure that the care and treatment is totally appropriate and that it allows choice and can be 'mixed and matched' according to need. The caring team must also offer support, explanation and companionship in a way that is acceptable to the patient and their family.

It is sometimes difficult, even for the most experienced nurse, to determine what in fact are the final hours and many patients who have appeared to be within 2–3 hours of death will survive for several more days.

Some terminally ill patients die suddenly from severe haemorrhage or pulmonary embolism and this can be very distressing. However, the majority gradually weaken as their vital functions become less able to cope. They then pass gently into unconsciousness and finally into respiratory or cardiac failure.

SIGNS OF APPROACHING DEATH

Nurses attending the patient throughout the 24 hours are often the first to observe changes that indicate impending death. Such changes can be summarized as follows.

1. There may be a gradual loss of interest in what is happening around them, but this is not universal and many patients retain their interest in life to the very end. Some patients are wanting to die and may appear to have 'given up' some while earlier.
2. Patients whose symptoms have so far been well controlled may become restless, agitated and obviously uncomfortable. They may start plucking at the bedclothes and a slight frown or tautness of the facial muscles may indicate the presence of underlying pain or discomfort. General weakness or drowsiness may prevent the patient from describing their problem. Pain may still be present, even if the patient is in coma, so analgesia should be maintained, but possibly at a reduced dose.
3. Mentally, patients may remain very alert until remarkably near the end and they may voice the knowledge of their impending death with incredible certainty. This may take the inexperienced nurse aback, but it is important to stay with the patient and allow the patient to talk it through, as frequently there is an accompanying fear of how death may finally come and what lies beyond.
4. Conversely, some patients pass through altered states of confusion, often due to biochemical changes or toxic effects of infection. However, anxiety and fear can play their part too and a calming, reassuring close relative is often the best person to assist the patient.
5. Patients become increasingly unwilling or unable to take food or fluids. The mouth is usually very dry, as at this stage patients frequently breathe through the mouth.
6. Changes in colour may occur, such as extreme pallor, cyanosis or jaundice. In these days, living in a multiracial society, it is essential to learn to observe the differences in colour that take place in those with non-white skins.
7. Changes in pulse rate and rhythm are important observations. The pulse may become weak, thready, rapid and irregular – it may no longer be felt at the wrist but have to be taken at the carotid artery in the neck or it may be necessary to feel for the heartbeat.

8. Changes in breathing are often a sign of impending death and can take various forms. Stridulous or noisy breathing, sometimes called the 'death rattle', is due to the accumulation of secretions in the larynx and trachea, which the patient is too weak to cough up. Air hunger – gasping for air – may be associated with internal haemorrhage and is also a very distressing sign. Cheyne–Stokes respirations involve periods of apnoea, followed by increasingly rapid respirations that reach a peak and then gradually become quieter until apnoea occurs again. This cycle is often repeated until breathing ceases for good. The jaw may droop or be tightly clenched. There may be hiccoughs due to uraemia.
9. The eyes may be staring, squinting or have a rather glazed look. When the fatty pads lining the eye socked have atrophied, due to wasting, there is a hollow-eyed appearance, which is very characteristic.

   Sometimes the eyes are closed, but they may remain open even when the patient is unconscious, which is rather distressing.
10. Due to relaxation of the sphincter muscles, incontinence of urine and/or faeces may occur. However, it is possible for retention and faecal impaction to be present and to cause restlessness.
11. Increasing coldness of the body may be observed, especially obvious in the limbs, together with mottling of the skin. A cold sweat may appear on the face and hands.
12. Altered states of consciousness are common; the patient may fail to respond to stimuli and then appear to regain some degree of response. Twitching, especially of limbs, may occur.

    Then, eventually there is a lapse into the coma preceding death.
13. The change in facial expression, from what may have been agonized and fearful to one of calmness and tranquillity in death, can be very striking and also very reassuring. The patient may also appear younger than in life as after a while lines disappear from the face and a smoothness is seen.

NURSING CARE

Whilst the following quotation is relevant to all aspects of management of the last hours, it is also very applicable to nursing care.

> Thou shalt not kill, but needst not strive officiously to keep alive.
> (Clough, 1961)

The care will make so much difference to the comfort of the dying patient and it must be carried out with great gentleness and understanding, the maintenance of dignity being of paramount importance. It is also of great benefit to the patient and the relatives if an atmosphere of calm, without a sense of hurry or 'busyness', can be maintained.

Where to nurse the patient is also of concern and it must be remembered that a single room and the ward area can both be lonely environments. There may be several reasons for considering it an advantage to nurse the patient in the single room, but again it must be based on individual need, the most likely being extreme confusion with restlessness, which can be distressing for other patients, or when it is difficult to control unpleasant odours. For some patients and their families, the lack of privacy in a ward may make a side room desirable, but isolation and unshared stress of relatives must be recognized and prevented.

Pain

As the patient's condition weakens it may be appropriate to reduce the dose of analgesia, especially if renal failure is apparent, but pain control is still very necessary. The administration of analgesia and other medication may now best be given by continuous subcutaneous injection via a Graseby syringe driver. This method avoids the need to disturb the patient too frequently and is also effective when swallowing and/or intestinal absorption is impaired.

Respiratory problems

The symptom known as 'the death rattle' has already been described. In the majority of cases this does not trouble the patient but the noise causes distress to the relatives and other patients in the ward. Changing the patient's position, for example from one side to another, may alleviate the problem. If not, drugs will be prescribed such as hyoscine or atropine. It is important to remember the side effects of these drugs and, therefore, not to give them before the terminal phase. However, at the same time they need to be given sooner rather than later, as they will be ineffective once the lungs are congested with fluid or the patient is in heart failure. If hyoscine is given for more than 24 hours, tolerance to it may develop rapidly and therefore the dose will almost certainly need to be increased. If there is some pulmonary oedema a diuretic such as frusemide will be given by injection. In extreme cases suction can be used, but this may cause distress to the patient and it must be done with extreme gentleness and skill.

Hygiene and comfort

Whilst it is essential that the patient is kept clean, dry and as comfortable as possible, it is necessary not to further exhaust them during the last hours by overzealous personal hygiene. The face, hands and genital area should be washed as appropriate. Actual sores and wounds will be dressed as necessary and particular care taken to try and lessen unpleasant odours, such as may be associated with fungating wounds or fistulae.

It is important to change the patient's position regularly and as necessary especially if breathing appears laboured or they seem uncomfortable. It is sometimes difficult to 'fix' the pillows, but time spent in the rearranging and the use of V-shaped pillows can make such a difference to comfort.

Pillows for the feet, bed cradles, loose clothing and little shawls are all aids to comfort. Recognition of the patient's sensations of cold or overheating is also vital.

When linen needs changing, and fresh bedlinen is essential, the use of a hoist may lessen the inevitable disturbance. Occasionally, a patient will prefer to rest in an armchair and may die peacefully in this position.

The use of pads may be appropriate when the patient is unable to use the commode and catheterization is inappropriate. They will also prevent excess soiling by faecal incontinence.

Nasal passages should be kept clear and nostrils free from any dried secretions. If necessary, cotton buds could be used. Additional eye care may be necessary to prevent discharge. Swabbing with normal saline should be adequate. Every effort should be made to keep the eyelids closed in unconscious patients.

Mouth care and oral fluids

As many patients breathe through the mouth at this stage and are often reluctant or unable to drink, the care of the mouth is of vital importance. A dry mouth adds to the patient's discomfort, so frequent attention is necessary.

A small, soft toothbrush may still be used, but foam sticks (sponges) dipped in a suitable oral solution may be better. Treatment must be carried out gently and with care, as some patients may bitterly resent such treatment and will resist and clench the teeth. Dentures should be removed if the patient is semiconscious. Lip salve can be applied to the lips.

Alternative means of taking small amounts of fluid which might be acceptable to the patient include:

- tiny ice chips, which can be fruit flavoured;
- ice lollies or soft fruit sweets to suck;
- tiny pieces of pineapple to chew;
- foam covered sticks dipped in a favourite fruit juice.

More active measures to provide fluid may cause added distress. In fact a slight degree of dehydration in a dying patient might be more comfortable, for example, leading to less urine output and fewer respiratory secretions. However, this does reinforce the importance of mouth care and perhaps raise the issue of adequate explanation of such management to the relatives and junior staff.

Restlessness

It is quite common for patients during the last hours of life to become increasingly restless. This can be distressing for the patient, but is probably more so for relatives and other patients. The grieving of relatives may be intensified if their last memories are those of a very restless loved one.

Every effort should therefore be made to try and discover the cause, despite the fact it may be a sign of impending death. With this in mind, it must be recognized that the patient may be unable to make their discomfort, pain or fears known. This may be due now to an inability to communicate by speech which is clear and coherent or because they have reverted to their mother tongue. It must also be remembered that the patient may not be using a hearing aid at this stage or wearing their dentures. All such problems will severely limit communication with carers.

The commonest and most easily rectified causes of restlessness may be a full bladder, a dry mouth, positional discomfort and pain. Whilst it should not occur at this stage, it is possible that severe constipation is also a cause.

The physical causes of restlessness mentioned above may be further identified by the patient appearing 'fidgety' and unable to find a comfortable position. Causes due to metabolic upset such as uraemia or to cerebral metastases or oedema or the withdrawal of some medications (especially if they cannot be taken orally and have not been given by another route such as the syringe driver) may be identified by uncontrollable twitchiness of the limbs – the 'restless legs' syndrome.

In some patients, the restlessness may be combined with confusion.

When all possible causes have been investigated and appropriate treatment tried, but without adequate effect, then sedation should be used. The use of midazolam, a water-soluble, short-acting benzodiazepine, does appear to be effective. It is a muscle relaxant and gives sedation with amnesia. Midazolam can be given subcutaneously via a syringe driver and can be combined with antiemetics and opioids.

Sudden death

There are a small minority who may die suddenly from a severe bleed such as haemoptysis, haematemesis or bleeding from an ulcerated/fungating wound. This is obviously extremely frightening for the patient and therefore they should never be left alone. These problems have been discussed in a previous chapter.

SPIRITUAL CARE

Throughout these last hours, the nurse's approach to the dying person must be one of care, support and sympathetic understanding, all shown as a respect of the individual human being, making every effort to maintain their dignity. As has been said, some patients are in a great fear and dread of death and have not come to terms with their illness.

They should never be left alone when their condition has deteriorated and death is expected soon. A relative, friend or nurse should be at the bedside and available to comfort and support the patient. One cannot stress too strongly the value of touch, which keeps dying individuals in contact with these around them: holding their hands, gently caressing their back and talking to them quietly all may help them in their last moments. One must always remember that hearing is the last sense lost and often patients can hear someone speaking even if they are apparently in a coma. The nurse should never say anything in the presence of the seemingly unconscious patient that would not be said to their face.

Religious and cultural aspects of care

In continuing to care for the dying patient as a unique person the nurse should recognize the particular importance for the patient and family of religious and cultural aspects during the last hours and at the moment of death. For the family, great importance may also be attached to ritual surrounding the funeral and throughout the period of mourning. It is considered that some measure of ritual helps the bereaved to come to terms gradually with the loss of their relative and a turning point in their own lives. Whether acknowledged or not, many rituals at this time have a religious element.

There is also the question of giving spiritual support to the large number of individuals in the UK who profess no particular faith, although it may have been assumed that they are nominal Christians. All these matters are considered in other chapters in relation to dying patients and their families, before the patient is actually near to death. The following section concentrates on care during the late stage of dying and immediately after death, with regard to some of the major world faiths.

The Christian faith

Practising Christians of all denominations will welcome the ministrations of a priest or minister when they are dying and the nurse should facilitate this, meeting any requests of the patient. There may be a situation where the relatives are not of the same denomination and tact is essential to avoid any conflict between their views and the clearly expressed wishes of the patient. When this seems likely, a team approach is advisable rather than the nurse trying to resolve the matter alone. If the particular church has a sacramental system, the patient is likely to have received the sacraments before death is imminent.

If the patient is dying at home and has one or more relatives, they will be the link between the patient and their religious minister and the nurse will simply ensure that there are no difficulties, for example, of communication, with the minister requested. Even so, the nurse might be present at the death and invited to share with the family in customary prayers at the bedside to console the dying person (who may still be able to hear) in their last moments. The prayers may be led by the priest or minister or by a member of the family or the nurse might be requested to read them.

In hospital or other institutions the nurse should ascertain whether the chaplain wishes to be called at the time of death. The chaplain's decision will depend on circumstances such as the closeness of the last visit and the wishes of the family. As at home, it is customary to recite short commendatory prayers for the consolation of the patient and family, if they are present.

Non-Christian faiths

Judaism

The saving of life because the body is considered 'the vessel of divine creation' is of the utmost importance to the Jew and this can, therefore, produce some conflict as the patient approaches death. However, with gentle skill and tact and the introduction of a rabbi, much can be done to help patients accept their situation and turn their eyes to the afterlife that their faith incorporates. Judaism does not define the form of this afterlife except for a belief in reward and punishment. The person near to death, therefore, is encouraged to recite the 'confession on the death-bed' and the words of the monotheistic declaration in the last verse of the Book of Deuteronomy – 'Hear O Israel, the Lord our God is one God' – should be the last words of the dying person, said for them if they are unable. The relatives or friends may wish to read scriptures or lamentations just after death and a single room may make this easier.

Islam

Muslims are urged to seek forgiveness and mercy from God and to affirm the unity of God before death, but they do not need any 'minister' to help in this matter. However, they will usually want the family or members of the local mosque to recite the holy book, *The Koran*, with them while they are dying. Allowing patients to face Mecca as they are dying is important to them. This means placing them on their right side with their face towards Mecca or on their back with their feet in the direction of Mecca and their head slightly raised so that they face it. 'There is no God but God and Muhammad is the Prophet of God' will be their last words or whispered into their ear by a member of the family. Sweet-smelling substances may be placed by the patient but any means of diversion such as music should be kept away from them. It is perhaps important for the nurse to realize that menstruating women and women during the 40-day period after childbirth are considered ritually impure and may, therefore, be kept away from the dying patient.

Hinduism

Hindus believe in reincarnation. A Hindu prepares for death by leading a calm life, by rejoicing in the things of the spirit and by being detached from all sensual pleasures. As Hindus are dying, money and clothes may be brought to them to touch before they are distributed to the poor. Some relatives or a priest will usually sit with them and read from a holy book, *The Bhagavadgita*. Sometimes the patient may wish to lie on the ground to be close to Mother Earth at the time of death, to have an oil lamp lit and incense burned. The eldest son will be expected to lead the family at this time and even if he is a small child he will be expected to be present before, during and after the death of his father. The families may often grieve aloud at the time of death, regarding this as a help and in no way unsuitable.

Sikhism

As the Sikh is dying, relatives and friends will read from the Sikh holy book, *Guru Granth Sahab*. Sikhs believe in reincarnation and this may make their actual death easier. The Sikhs do not permit loud lamentations at the time of death but are likely to exclaim 'Wahiguru, Wahiguru' ('Wonderful Lord').

Buddhism

Buddhists also believe in reincarnation. Sickness and death are very much accepted as part and parcel of life. Death should be a calm affair and therefore those present may use a text that will induce equanimity and fortitude. A Buddhist monk should be informed as soon after death as possible so that he may perform the necessary prayers that may take about an hour. However, these prayers do not need to be said over the body but may be said in a temple at some distance away.

Nurses should take the trouble to inform themselves regarding the religious and cultural background of each individual patient and their family, so as to be able to give the maximum help and support at this critical time.

CARE OF THE FAMILY

Although the nurse will take a close interest in the welfare of the relatives of the dying patient from the beginning of their relationship, this reaches its climax during the last hours of a patient's life. The circumstances will be variable. For instance, the dying process may have been a comparatively long one, so the family may have become very tired under the strain either of caring for the patient at home or making frequent journeys to hospital or hospice. If the terminal illness has advanced rapidly, the patient may be admitted for residential care, literally within the last hours of life.

'Family' may consist of a large number of people of different degrees of kinship, all anxious to do the right thing for a loved member. At the other end of the scale, there may be only one close relative or just a close friend. It is appropriate to remember here the special and sometimes difficult situation for the partner of a dying person in a homosexual relationship who wishes to keep vigil at the bedside during the last hours. Those gathered at the bedside may not always be a united, loving family – either among themselves or in their relationship with the dying patient. Because of the variability of the situation, the nurse may be supporting the family in a peaceful atmosphere or one charged with emotional tension. Nurses need to have a calm, sensitive approach themselves, realizing that conflicting feelings may sometimes cause relatives to act in a way that seems unreasonable and difficult to help.

Cultural background also plays a part. It has been noted that those holding a non-Christian religious faith (predominantly from the Asian continent) may be uninhibited in outward manifestation of grief. The Latin races also have a tendency to this characteristic, as also do Jewish people. In contrast, the British traditional reserve, especially in men, may result in silent, tearless grief, none the less agonizing for that.

Practical help for the family

1. It is the right of the close family members to come and go as they please, whether it is day or night. If there are several relatives, they

may wish to provide a continuous rota so that the patient is never left alone. If this is not possible a nurse should sit with the patient at the intervening times. In any case, the nurse should come frequently to observe the patient and do anything that is required for their comfort, involving a relative if they wish in such actions as moistening the patient's lips. To leave the relatives alone for too long adds to their anxiety and possible fear of the impending death.

2. Any information that the relatives request should be readily given by the nurse and the doctor. It should be made clear that the patient is expected to die within the next few hours, but that no-one can predict the exact time. If the relatives decide to leave the bedside it should be established whether they wish to be present when the patient dies and how quickly they can be contacted.
3. Some provision should be made for a relative to rest at intervals – provide a comfortable armchair next to the bed or a couch of some kind and facilities in a room near to the patient. Relatives need some light nourishment; even if not hungry, cups of tea or coffee are welcome. Those who are smokers should be able to indulge at this time, without disapproval, away from the patient's bedside.
4. Whatever is wished by the family (and presumed to be the wish of the patient) regarding religious ministrations should be carried out, as described earlier in this chapter.
5. Relatives will appreciate the reassurance that the patient is being kept free from pain and to witness concern for their comfort. The patient may remain conscious almost to the end, although the majority lapse into coma at some point during the last hours. It is helpful to explain that even an apparently unconscious patient may still be able to hear and a reassuring squeeze given, showing that they are not alone.

Younger colleagues, student nurses or nursing auxiliaries need the support of the trained nurse if they have never witnessed the last hours of a dying patient and the death itself. They need to participate in the care of both the patient and the family both for their own development and to learn how to give these last services.

THE MOMENT OF DEATH

Where there has been a gradual progression towards death, there will be progressive dysfunction of one or more of the major systems of the body. Death will be recognized by the cessation of respiration and of the heart-beat (which may sometimes be present even when no pulse can be found at the wrist). The pupils of the eyes will be fixed and dilated and the skin of the face and extremities feels very cold to the touch.

The time of death should be noted and the doctor who has been treating the patient informed, as they must subsequently certify the death. Although the doctor must have seen the patient prior to death, there is no legal requirement that they must view the body after death.

In the case of sudden and unexpected death, e.g. due to head injury or cerebral anoxia from cardiac arrest, a doctor must be sent for immediately who will wish to satisfy themselves that, as well as the classic signs of cessation of respiration and heartbeat, there is also total and irreversible loss of brainstem function.

Immediate needs

As soon as the patient has died, the relatives should be allowed to remain with the deceased for a short while in privacy. A nurse should then gently escort them to a room away from the bedside, whilst two other nurses straighten the limbs of the dead body, ensuring the eyes are closed and leaving the bed and surroundings clean and tidy, remembering that some relatives may want to return for a final farewell.

In the meantime, the relatives should be given the opportunity to be alone together for a time, the nurse returning with a tray of tea and a sympathetic presence. It is essential to explain to the bereaved that it is perfectly natural in such circumstances to cry and be upset: it is part of the pattern of bereavement and is to be expected. Some relatives may experience feelings of guilt or relief from strain and may act in totally unpredictable ways that may be somewhat disturbing. The nurse should not appear to be upset by this, but allow the individuals to get rid of their tensions in any way they like and just to be there to offer help.

Sometimes the nurse may also be particularly moved by the patient's death and share in the grief of the relatives in a spontaneous expression of emotion such as putting their arms around a relative and shedding a few tears. This demonstration of closeness is often very comforting to the family, but naturally this must be combined with the nurse continuing in their role of supporter in a calm and capable manner. There may also be less experienced young colleagues who need an example and help in coping with their own emotions whilst caring for the family.

Before leaving, the relatives should have been given clear information regarding the collection of the death certificate and the personal belongings of the deceased the next day. If any social problems are likely to occur as a result of the death, the relatives will have been referred to the social worker, who will be able to give help and advice. If additional support is necessary, as in the case of a father left with young children or an elderly person left without relatives or those for whom the death has presented complicated psychological problems, a bereavement team is valuable, offering regular visits and the use of their skills to assist in every way possible.

Sudden and unexpected death

The family of a person who dies quite unexpectedly, having last been seen apparently fit and well, are likely to pass through a series of severe reactions. At first there will be bewilderment and failure to comprehend what has happened, followed by a state of shock. The deceased person may have been found dead at home or brought to a hospital already dead.

The relatives will need treating with gentleness and compassion and should not be left alone. A friend or less involved member of the family who can give warm but calm support will be a great asset to the nurse in their efforts to support the relatives at this initial stage. There may be uncontrollable crying or a feeling of numbness and unreality. Later the relatives will want to talk about the situation with the doctor and nurse and ask questions about the circumstances of the death. They are likely to ask to see the body and should be prepared for any possibly distressing features.

One of the most tragic situations is if the deceased person has committed suicide, without any apparent prior intimation of this. Inevitably the family will question whether they are to blame and could have done anything to avert the tragedy. They will need to talk about their feelings and their deceased relative and need long term professional support during the process of mourning. In all these distressing situations, careful explanations must be given in simple terms and in an unhurried way.

LAST OFFICES

In judging when to commence Last Offices, it should be remembered that rigor mortis (contraction of muscles) generally appears 2–4 hours after death, attaining its full intensity within 48 hours and disappearing within another 48 hours.

Last Offices have always been recognized as the final service offered as a mark of respect to the dead person before burial or cremation. Again, it is important to be sensitive to the beliefs of the family as to how Last Offices are carried out. In some instances, the nurse will play no part as the family will do all that they wish. In the case of Christians or those of no particular religious faith, two nurses should carry out the following actions, unless the undertaker is to do all or most of these:

1. The body is washed and dressed in a shroud, clean nightdress/pyjamas or clothing requested by the relations.

2. Catheters and other appliances (syringe drivers) are removed and any sores and wounds sealed with a waterproof dressing. Safety pins are not used.
3. Body orifices may be packed.
4. The lower jaw may need to be supported with a bandage, in order to keep the mouth closed. Dentures, if worm, should be replaced in the mouth if possible (consent of relatives might need to be sought).
5. Rings and other jewellery are usually removed and returned to relatives.
6. An identity label, giving the patient's full name and registration number, should be attached to the ankle (identity labels already in position should be left). It is insufficient to mark only the outside of the shroud.

Some families may wish to have a favourite object left with the body although this is often discussed later with the undertaker rather than at this stage. For some, a religious memento is important and for some Roman Catholic families a crucifix or rosary may be placed in the hands of the dead person. The body may be taken to a chapel of rest where the relatives can see it before the undertakers remove it. The body will usually remain at the undertakers until the funeral takes place; sometimes in the Roman Catholic Church the body will lie in the church the night preceding the funeral. This also occurs in the Eastern Orthodox Churches, the only difference being that here the body may be in an open coffin. Burial or cremation is acceptable to all.

Judaism

'Progressive' or 'Liberal' Jews may permit the body to be laid out in the normal way by the nurses. However, many will join their Orthodox co-religionists in requiring a strict ritual. The nurse must discover beforehand what will be required. For the Orthodox Jew, the nurse may straighten the body, close the eyes, place the arms straight down the side of the body and bandage the jaw. Any intravenous infusion or drainage tubes are removed and the body is then wrapped in a plain white sheet before being taken from the ward. Some may require that the nurse wears disposable gloves to carry out the above.

A 'watcher' may be designated from the family or local synagogue to remain with the body until burial, although this is often waived in large hospitals as they feel there is always someone in attendance. However, if this is the case, facilities should be made available and the use of a viewing room may be helpful. The body is washed by members of an appointed burial society; men wash men and women wash women. There are usually three present and prayers are said at the same time. This may take place in the hospital mortuary. There is no embalming, preservatives or cosmetics are not used and the body is placed in a plain white shroud in a plain coffin. The burial usually takes place within 24 hours of death after a short half-hour burial service. The family follow this by a strict seven days of mourning and prayers. Reform Jews may occasionally desire cremation.

The body is regarded by Jews as God's gift and therefore they do not accept post-mortems unless legally required. They will donate organs but only on complete death and not 'clinical death' and only when the prospective operation is well enough established to offer good prognosis to the recipient, i.e. it is well beyond the experimental stage.

Islam

Muslims also have strict washing rituals and these are usually performed by a member of the family designated by the deceased or, if not, the closest relative. Disposable gloves must be used by the nurse, who is permitted to straighten the body, bandage the jaw and remove drainage tubes, etc. After the washing, Muslim men are wrapped in three cloths and women in five cloths and once completed, burial is urged without delay. Cremation is strictly forbidden and if at all possible burial should take place within a Muslim burial ground. In the country of origin, no coffins are permitted, but must be used in Britain. The body is laid on its right side so that it faces Mecca.

Post-mortems are forbidden unless legally required and then careful explanation will be needed. Organ donation is also strictly forbidden.

Hinduism

Some Hindu families will not follow any specific Last Offices and the nurses can proceed as usual. However, for others, the relatives will perform the duties led by the eldest son. The body is dressed in new clothes before it leaves the hospital. A Hindu woman wears a marriage cord around her neck and this must only be cut after her death and only by her husband. It is perhaps a sensitive gesture for the nurse to ask for this to be done before a post-mortem, should one take place. Again, Hindus will only accept post-mortems if they are legally required and even then great sensitivity must be shown and many feel it is repugnant, showing no respect for the dead person to gain peace in the next life.

Cremation is preferred by Hindus and traditionally the eldest son lights the funeral pyre. However, this is forbidden in Britain, so Hindus here have developed symbolic gestures to fulfil this duty. Children under five, however, are buried.

Sikhism

Last Offices are usually performed by the family but the nurse must ask if they wish to do so in this country. The nurse may close the eyes, straighten the limbs and wrap the body in a sheet. If the nurse has been allowed to perform the Last Offices it must be remembered that the Sikh is cremated wearing the five 'K' symbols.

Buddhism

There are no specific Last Offices for Buddhists and therefore the nurse can proceed as usual. Helping others is central to their philosophy so there will be no objection to organ transplants. In some countries cremation is the accepted practice, but the Buddhist family may be more flexible in Britain. Committal depends on the lunar calendar and may be within 3–7 days. A Buddhist monk will usually be called for the funeral and it tends to be a solemn affair reflecting the sadness of the human loss.

Removal of the body

If the patient dies in an institution, the body will need to be removed from the ward or room after Last Offices have been performed. The nurse has a responsibility to ensure that this is done in a dignified way, not least for the sake of other patients who may be aware of what is happening.

Sometimes relatives may arrive later and wish to pay their last respects. It is helpful if a room is available adjoining the mortuary for this purpose unless the relatives can say farewell in the ward before the body is removed. They will need the same support and sympathetic handling as for relatives present at the time of death.

STAFF SUPPORT

Nurses who have not been present at a death before may feel rather nervous and anxious at such a time, not knowing what to expect or what to do, and a senior nurse should do all that is possible to guide them practically, to help them understand their feelings, to realize that death comes to us all – that it is a fact we must learn to live with. It should be stressed that by acting in a positive manner with the dying patient and by using their nursing skills, they enable the patient to die comfortably. Appreciating the place of prayer at the time of death will enable them to see beyond the event. Helping them to see the needs of the family for comfort and support at this time will aid nurses in overcoming any anxiety. Taking the new nurse outside and explaining 'Last Offices' to them and taking them through it practically, showing respect for the body in gentle and sensitive handling, may all make it into a positive experience, again enabling the nurse to come to terms with death.

The senior nurse should also be aware that many young nurses suffer delayed reactions. They may become quiet or emotional over something quite unrelated. Others may not show anything, but it is important that all are given the chance to talk when they need a listening ear. A general atmosphere of caring for each other does much to enable more junior staff to voice their problems over particular deaths.

In hospice wards, a number of deaths in a short space of time can become difficult for all members of staff and then it can be helpful for both senior and junior nurses to sit down together and talk over a cup of tea. Regular interdisciplinary staff meetings can also be helpful as a means of supporting one another. For any nurse working fulltime in the field of terminal care, an active social life should be encouraged.

LEGAL ASPECTS

Nurses need to know the principles of the legal aspects involved just before and after the death of a patient. They may be asked questions by the relatives and should be able to answer them.

Next-of-kin

It is very important to establish who is next-of-kin and where they may be contacted. One would think this was an easy task but it is not always so, as one discovers through bitter experience. For example, two ladies may claim to be the wife of the patient or a hitherto unknown relative may turn up and insist that he or she is next-of-kin. Much tact is needed to deal with such situations.

Time of death

The exact time of death should be noted and the doctor, if not present, should be informed who was present at the time of death. The names of those present are recorded, both relatives and staff.

Last Offices

As already mentioned above, the relatives' wishes must be ascertained to avoid possible future litigation as well as natural distress. If there is any question of criminal proceedings there should be minimal interference with the body.

Property of the deceased patient

Any valuables or large sums of money should already have been deposited for safe keeping with the hospital administrator and the nearest relative can collect them when convenient. Other belongings normally kept in the bedside locker should be listed by two nurses who then sign the list as a correct record. The property is packed into a parcel or box and may be given to the relatives at a suitable moment, usually when they come for the death certificate.

Existence of a valid will

Nurses may be questioned regarding the advisability of making a will and should encourage all patients who are terminally ill to do so, as this prevents much friction and even family feuds after the death. If, however, they are asked to act as witnesses to a patient's will, they are well advised not to do so but to suggest that a solicitor should see the patient and find witnesses. At the same time as this is drawn up, the doctor has to write a statement in the case notes about the patient's mental state in case the will is later contested.

As a valuable document, the will can then be deposited for safe keeping with the hospital administrator, if this is what the patient desires. The hospice/hospital social worker is also likely to be involved with this aspect.

Death certificate

If the cause of death is clear and there are no suspicious circumstances, the doctor caring for the patient will sign the death certificate and arrangements can be made for the relatives to collect this and take it to the registrar as soon as possible. If cremation is to take place, the law requires a further certificate signed by two doctors.

Donation of organs for transplant or research

The nearest relative must act quickly if this was the wish of the deceased person; kidneys must be removed within half an hour of death, eyes within six hours. The nurse's involvement in this matter will consist of making sure that the relatives are in touch with the doctor concerned and in being aware that, as with a request for a post-mortem examination or a coroner's inquest, this can add to distress and increase the need for support at this time.

ACKNOWLEDGEMENTS

We acknowledge the help of the Islamic Foundation in Leicester and the Buddhist Society in London.

We also acknowledge the work in the previous edition by Sister Marcella Cassells and Bernadette Ross.

REFERENCES

Clough, A. (1961) The Latest Decalogue, in *Penguin Dictionary of Quotations*, (eds M.J. Cohen and J.M. Cohen), Penguin, Harmondsworth.

Twycross, R.G. (1984) *A Time to Die*, CMF Publications, London, p. 10.

Twycross, R. G. (1986) *The Dying Patient*, CMF Publications, London, p. 7.

FURTHER READING

Baqui, M.A., Joseph, Rabbi B. and Levenstein, Rabbi M. (1983) *Jewish and Muslim Teaching Concerning Death*, St Joseph's Hospice, London.

Baqui, M.A., Joseph, Rabbi B. and Levenstein, Rabbi M. (1993) *Our Ministry and Other Faiths – A Booklet for Hospital Chaplains*, CIO Publishing, London.

Bassett, C. (1993) The living will – implications for nurses. *British Journal of Nursing*, **2**(13), 688–91.

Black, I. (1992) Terminal restlessness in patients with advanced malignant disease. *Journal of Palliative Medicine*, **6**(4), 293–8.

Centre for Medical Education (1992) *Helpful Essential Links to Palliative Care*, University of Dundee and Cancer Relief Macmillan Fund.

Church Pastoral Aid Society Adult Training & Resources (1993) *Living with Loss*, CPAS, Warwick.

Dicks, B. (1990) The contribution of nursing to palliative care. *Journal of Palliative Medicine*, **4**, 197–203.

Green, J. (1991) *Death with Dignity – Meeting Spiritual Needs of Patients in a Multicultural Society*, Nursing Times Book Service, Macmillan, Basingstoke.

Hanratty, J. (1983) *Care of the Dying – Philosophy of the Care of the Terminally Ill*, St Joseph's Hospice, London.

Hanratty, J. (1985) *The Physiology of Dying*, St Joseph's Hospice, London.

Hanratty, J. (1987) *Control of Distressing Symptoms in the Dying Patient*, St Joseph's Hospice, London.

Henley, A. (1979) *Asian Patients in Hospital and at Home*, King Edward's Hospital Fund for London.

House, N. (1993) Helping to reach an understanding – palliative care for people from ethnic minority groups. *Professional Nurse*, **8**(5), 329–32.

Irvine, B. (1993) Developments in palliative nursing in and out of the hospital setting. *British Journal of Nursing*, **2**(4), 218–24.

Lothian Community Relations Council (1984) *Religious Cultures*, LCRC, Edinburgh.

McGilloway, O. and Myco, F. (eds) (1985) *Nursing and Spiritual Care*, Harper and Row, London.

McNamara, P., Minton, M. and Twycross, R. (1991) Use of midazolam in palliative care. *Journal of Palliative Medicine*, **5**(3), 244–9.

Penn, K. (1992) Passive euthanasia in palliative care. *British Journal of Nursing*, **1**(9), 462–6.

Prickett, J. (1980) *Death*, Living Faiths series, Butterworth Educational, Cambridge.

Rea, K. (1993) (Editorial) Who has the right to end life? *British Journal of Nursing*, **2**(6), 303.

Sampson, C. (1982) *The Neglected Ethic – Religious and Cultural Factors in the Care of Patients*, McGraw-Hill, Maidenhead.

Young, A.P. (1989) *Legal Problems in Nursing Practice*, 2nd edn, Harper and Row, London.

7 The role of the doctor

Let us begin with a paradox: doctors trained to cure, care for the incurable dying. Is this simply a recipe for frustration and failure for both the doctor and ill person or does this point to something deeper in the relationship between clinician and patient? To examine this question we will consider what defines a doctor, what roles they play and how the person behind these masks is the true source from which effective care for the dying is derived.

DEFINITIONS

The roots of words used to describe doctors (Hanks, 1986) throw some light on their roles:

Doctor: from *docere* (L) meaning 'to teach'

At first sight, this seems a surprising derivation for someone in the business of curing. Consider, however, the time spent talking to the dying person and his family about the illness, its treatment and prognosis, not to mention the teaching of other health care professionals. Further, in a counselling context, the doctor is helping patients to understand themselves better.

Physician: from *phusis* (Gk) meaning 'nature'

We all originate from the natural world. Many of our treatments come from nature, as with morphine which is derived from the opium poppy. Every therapy we use takes advantage of the natural healing processes of the body, such as after surgery. Death itself is a natural process which may be put off for many years but must happen eventually and it is part of the physician's work to look after the dying.

Healer: from *haelen* (Old English) meaning 'whole'

Defining health is like trying to hold a bar of wet soap – it keeps slipping out of your grasp. However, it does imply a person whose body, mind and spirit are in harmony both within the individual and in relating to the environment. Healing, then, means reuniting some aspect of the sick person which has become, so to speak, split off from the rest; in other words, to make whole again. Hence a holistic approach to medicine is rightly highly valued in palliative care. It might be argued, though, that someone dying of cancer can never be healed. This is contradicted by Stephen Levine (1987) describing patients who, even though they were dying, felt they had been healed in a way that accepted their illness and imminent death. More obviously, there may be healing of family relationships, of the psyche and of the spirit in parallel with advancing cancer.

The American slang 'medic' comes from the Latin *mederi*, also meaning 'to heal'.

Healing is not confined to doctors. This is especially true with the dying where relatives, friends, nurses, chaplains, physiotherapists, social workers, counsellors, volunteers and others may all bring healing and may often be more important in this process than the doctor.

Clinician: from *kline* (Gk) meaning 'bed'

The stereotype is so familiar – doctors dressed in white coats and stethoscopes stand around a sick person in bed. Why, though, is 'bed' automatically prescribed even before a patient enters a hospital or hospice? There are several factors; rest facilitates recovery; lying still allows wounds to heal; beds are safe places in an unfamiliar environment and define the ill person's own territory; and often the dying are simply too weak to get up, so that staying in bed acknowledges this necessary dependence. It is doubly important in the last case to ensure that autonomy is preserved as far as possible.

Therapist: from *therapeueim* (Gk) meaning 'to minister to'

This description is not specific to doctors but is included because of the important part actions play in the work of the doctor, even with the dying where, for example, surgery is usually no longer useful. The four main modes are communication (such as giving information or counselling), touch (as when the patient is examined), prescribing medicines (as with the vital role morphine plays in pain control) and procedures (for example, pleural taps). There is an often unrecognized ritual healing aspect to these actions which increases their power. An example is the placebo effect which has been described as the body's self-healing response (Reilly, personal communication).

It has been the author's experience in facilitating doctors' seminars on communication with the dying that it is when there are no more things to do that doctors feel most uncomfortable and distressed. Their roles have gone; they are left with themselves as people facing another person in pain and they cannot immediately make it better.

ROLES

At first sight it may seem that doctors have one role only – being doctors. Further thought, however, will show that they assume multiple roles and are also seen by others in various guises, some real, some imaginary, some benign and some malign (Table 7.1).

Assagioli (cited in Ferrucci, 1982) has called such roles subpersonalities, that is, constellations of behaviour patterns. These pertain to everyone; examples are the Judge, the Victim, the Child or the Wise Old Man. The essential point is that doctors should not become unconsciously trapped in them but are able to move in and out of those that are useful and avoid those that are not.

The doctor as clinician

Palliative care doctors do not have the satisfaction of healing their patients physically, so they cannot hide behind cures to avoid coming into

Table 7.1 Examples of real and illusory doctors' roles

Clinician	**Helper**	**Teamwork**
Healer	Comforter	Administrator
Symptomatologist	Friend	Manager
Surgeon	Supporter	Leader
Diagnostician	Psychotherapist	Team member
Pharmacologist	Guide	Colleague
Thanatologist	Enabler	Politician
Scientist	Burnt out	Apprentice
Education	**Spiritual**	**Blame**
Teacher	Priest	Scapegoat
Counsellor	Magician	Betrayer
Parent	Miracle worker	Experimenter
Writer	Prophet	Cold
Problem solver	God	Mechanic
Student		Inquisitor
		Judge

relationship with the terminally ill. They may of course have other defences such as dealing only with symptoms or being so busy with administration that they have little time to see patients. In practice, however, doctors wishing to work in palliative care will tend to bee those who value the personal aspect of medicine highly and so give priority to relating well to the ill person.

In the main, terminal care services in Great Britain and Ireland have focused on advanced cancer. Some also look after patients with motor neurone disease or chronic illnesses such as multiple sclerosis. More recently, help for HIV related illness has often been offered and there are now specialized units in this field such as the Mildmay Mission Hospital. Unfortunately, this is not yet the case for the large number of people dying of non-malignant diseases such as end-stage respiratory failure.

It might be thought that diagnosis goes out of the window in terminal care; after all, isn't advancing cancer, for example, obvious? Diagnosis still needs to be precise but is much more focused on problems as the patient sees them, such as causes of symptoms or reasons for family disharmony. This avoids the automatic response of: terminal cancer equals pain equals morphine and so on to the next patient.

Careful listening is, of course, essential in elucidating causes of symptoms, but will also be therapeutic in itself. The same applies to examination of the patient. Investigations are burdensome and only to be carried out if they will be of help towards symptom control.

Cicely Saunders (Saunders and Sykes, 1993) has rightly pointed out the manifold nature of suffering in the dying and has coined the phrase 'total pain' to describe not only physical but also mental, social and spiritual pain. Attention must be paid to all these aspects, otherwise, for example, unrelieved depression will make accompanying physical pain more resistant to treatment. Clearly, then, a holistic approach to therapy is essential.

Symptom control is one of the cornerstones of good palliative medicine. Patients in severe pain which occupies all their attention will not be able to talk about their worries concerning dying until they are relieved of their physical distress. Pain control, with figures quoted of 95% of patients obtaining effective alleviation (Takeda, 1986), has been one of the success stories of medicine in recent years and has done much to relieve the dark fears around the taboo subject of dying. The terminal care doctor, then, needs to be an expert clinical pharmacologist.

They particularly need to be discriminating in the use of drugs. Multiple symptoms beget polypharmacy; this is to some extent inevitable, but the difficulty that very frail patients have in swallowing all the pills prescribed invites ruthless pruning of the drug charts. The recent rapid growth in the use of the syringe driver has therefore been a great boon.

In the same way, use of medical procedures needs to be evaluated carefully. Urinary catheterization and enemas are obviously helpful, but other procedures such as transfusions or pleural taps do not necessarily improve symptoms and others such as gastrostomies or tracheostomies may sometimes leave the patient worse off than before.

Often symptom control is straightforward provided that there is attention to detail and frequent reassessment; the basics of regular analgesia given before the pain returns and in a dose sufficient to relieve the pain will still deal with most cases.

This is the cake on which the icing is the recent advances such as slow-release morphine or coeliac plexus blockade for upper abdominal pain due to malignancy.

One of the commonest questions the doctor is asked is 'how long?'. Doctors are in fact often inaccurate in their assessments of prognosis and, if anything, overestimate (Heyse-Moore and Johnson-Bell, 1987), despite the tendency of the patient and family to assign them prophetic powers. To the author's mind, therefore, the best answer is almost always 'I don't know'. This prevents the ill person or those close to them making plans on wrong information. An important exception is when the patient is within a day or two of death and the family want to sit with them overnight; or if a relative abroad is planning to come over at the end – in this case it is better to arrive too early rather than too late.

The doctor as helper

This role overlaps with that of clinician.

In medical school, cure is still often taught as the goal of all medical care and with this the unconscious and thus usually unchallenged assumption that people go on being 'cured' and hence go on living ad infinitum. This sets up the future doctor to fail.

It is important, therefore, to go back to the original motivation of medical students to become doctors. This surely is the care that one human being feels for another. Without this, doctors descend to being just cold mechanics. With this, all the skills developed, such as surgery, pharmacological expertise or psychotherapy, are simply ways of expressing their compassion. This may sound embarrassing – it would be so much easier to talk about interest in developments in medical technology, for example – but it is surely essential to stay in touch with this source, particularly in working with the dying. The question then becomes not 'How can I put this "body as a machine" right?' but rather, 'What does this ill person need?'. This avoids the frustration of preconceptions about what the doctor 'ought' to be doing and gives freedom to be creative and innovative in providing care.

Autonomy for the patient must be a prime concern here; this involves helping the ill person to help themselves and so feel in control where possible, but not expecting too much either. It is most important not to dictate to the patient; it is, after all, their illness. Further, collusion with the family in hiding the diagnosis from the patient must be avoided; they have a right to know if they wish and a right to honest answers to their questions. They also need the safety of knowing that information will not be forced on them before they are ready.

In all this, the doctor needs to create a safe space for the patient to talk freely, neither getting too close nor being too far away, neither being overwhelmed by the patient's distress nor appearing distant and uninterested. This benefits the doctor as well as the patient, since both over- and underinvolvement are stressful in their own ways. The middle way can allow the doctor to experience feelings in talking to the ill person and even to express them if this would be of help.

Clearly, then, counselling skills are an important part of the doctor's helping role, but must serve the underlying motivation of care, not be a substitute; a mechanical 'reflect the question', for example, will get nowhere. Problem solving skills, helping the patient to express feelings and come to an acceptance of their condition and providing emotional support are high priorities.

The way the doctor communicates with the dying person is not the regular hour a week of orthodox counselling; it could not be, since so many of the patients are within a week or two of dying. Instead, the time given to the patient may be only a few minutes or may be well over an hour. The ill person may want to talk at length several times a day or prefer to leave a week's gap in between conversations about their condition. They may wish to talk in depth to several different members of staff from different disciplines. Hence, it is vital to ensure that all such discussions are communicated to the other members of the multidisciplinary team.

The same considerations apply for the family. Sometimes they need more time than the patient. Seeing the family together as much as possible, along with the patient where appropriate, will avoid being caught up in family conflicts and ensure that communication is first hand, rather than reported, with all its attendant potential for inaccuracies of information.

Helping the dying in this way can be stressful to the doctor. They have to accept their own pain at seeing someone suffer and their powerlessness at not being able to cure them. They will experience their own sense of loss when a patient they have befriended dies. Not surprisingly, then, burnout is an issue in terminal care. It is not an ideal term since the word seems to suggest an irreversible process. Perhaps a forest fire is a better metaphor since, although at first it seems as though the woods are completely destroyed, very soon the green shoots of new life appear. In practice, then, it is very important for the doctor to have their own support systems such as friends outside work, leisure pursuits, taking holidays and so on.

Teamwork

All clinical disciplines contribute to good palliative care. Hence, a multidisciplinary approach is essential, implying good communication and cooperation rather than competition and power struggles. It also means valuing and respecting the skills of each discipline.

In particular, the doctor–nurse relationship is crucial. The nurses are constantly on the ward and hence most closely in touch with any changes in the patient's condition. In this way, the doctor depends on the nurse. Further, although it is the doctor who prescribes, it is the nurse whose skill during the medicine rounds makes the giving of a certain drug feasible or who is best placed to decide, for example, that a change to a syringe driver is needed.

Receiving a report in the morning from the ward nurse and reporting back after the round or after seeing a new patient may seem very obvious ways for the doctor to communicate properly, but how often they are missed!

When dealing with families, it may be useful for the doctor to see them together with the nurse or social worker. This permits a synergistic pooling of expertise, allows staff to support each other during difficult interviews and saves time in avoiding needless repetition of family meetings with separate disciplines.

The doctor is often the leader in hospices, although there is no reason why this has to be so. It may be due to the way society views the doctor as a powerful figure able to cure lethal diseases and also to the competitiveness of getting into medical school which will tend to favour the more assertive students. Contrariwise, in some hospices, the nurse or the administrator is in charge.

In the business world, the managing director as dictator is a familiar caricature. This should not apply in palliative care where there is a very diverse group of disciplines which tends to favour a cooperative approach working by negotiation, not a feudal hierarchy. The leader, then, doctor or otherwise, guides and facilitates this process. Of course, managing conflict and the confrontations that may accordingly be necessary is also part of this role.

Doctors in hospices are, as much as their hospital colleagues, cursed with endless note taking and administration. A special factor is the very large number of death certificates and cremation papers needing completion, usually daily. A good working relationship with the local coroner and coroner's office is therefore a priority, especially, for example, where asbestos related disease is suspected and a post-mortem is mandatory.

Notifying the general practitioner the same working day that their patient has died or been discharged is not only courteous but important practically in ensuring that the patient has immediate medical support at home or that a bereaved relative is not left isolated.

The role of home care doctors varies somewhat from the above in that, when they visit, this is often alone and so they may have to become more directly involved in non-medical problems and ensuring that requests for help are passed to the appropriate team member. Good communication with the patient's general practitioner is essential as it is they who remain in charge and the home care doctor is there to advise them. In those domiciliary teams where there is an on-call service, the home care clinician may find, too, that they are called to confirm death and, as part of this, spend time comforting the bereaved relatives, help to lay the body out and advise about death certificates and undertakers.

The doctor as educator

Perhaps the most important educative role of the doctor is giving information to patients and their families. Often, breaking bad news leads to considerable emotional distress which means that very little is taken in by the ill person. So, saying only one thing at a time, leaving pauses, checking that the patient has understood, repeating what has been said as often as necessary, avoiding jargon and empathizing are all part of communicating well.

Another aspect is helping patients to clarify how they see their problems and what they can do towards solving them; this aids in preserving their autonomy and gives them some sense of control at a time of crisis when it seems that events are rapidly spiralling downhill and they feel powerless to do anything. A paraplegic patient, for example, who lives alone may think that even though they want to go home, it would be impossible because of their disability. However, by involving community support services, by asking relatives to stay at the patient's home if feasible, by bringing in the home care team and with the help of the hospice ambulance, what was a pipedream can suddenly become reality.

Hospices manage 5–15% of cancer deaths, depending on locality in Britain. Clearly, then, passing on the expertise developed in palliative care centres to those health care professionals looking after the other 85% or more is vital in ensuring high standards of terminal care in the community and in hospital. So, educational opportunities must be seized, whether through invitations to give talks outside the hospice or by creating teaching events inhouse. Many medical schools still only allocate a few hours in a five year syllabus specifically for teaching palliative medicine; hence medical students need to be prime targets for education in this area.

In all this, high teaching standards are a must. Good education is not like filling an empty pot but more like how children build a Lego set (Coles, 1989). Participative teaching methods using role play, group discussion or guided imagery, for example, may be more appropriate in teaching communication skills with the dying than a standard lecture format.

The doctor and spirituality

Despite the projections sometimes placed on them by patients and their families, doctors are not miracle workers, prophets or magicians; nor are they God. Doctors are given considerable respect by society and perhaps few are humble enough to avoid taking on to some degree the above-mentioned roles. The autocratic consultant surgeon is a familiar stereotype.

Doctors are subject to illusions of immortality, just like everyone else, and need to remember, especially in working with the dying, that the truth is otherwise:

> Like all the others, I too am a mortal
>   person . . .
> I too, when I was born, drew in the common air,
> I fell on the same ground that bears us all,
>   a wail my first sound . . .
> for all there is only one way into life, as out
>   of it.
>
> (*Wisdom 7:1–6*)

Some dying people are desperate to try anything in the faint hope of a cure and are therefore prepared to put their faith in the doctor, trying even experimental forms of, for example, chemotherapy despite the chances of a remission being almost nil. Clearly, it is necessary for the doctor to resist the temptation to go along with this if they feel such therapy won't work.

With the decreased practice of organized religion in the Western world, the doctor is sometimes cast as substitute for the priest. While this is, of course, not their role, especially if the sacramental aspect of the priesthood is considered, there is a way in which all clinical workers in palliative care, including doctors, have a pastoral function. This is to do with helping the ill person, if they so wish, to get in touch with their innermost essence, that which has deepest meaning for them, whether this be seen as the soul and hence God for those who have a belief or the individual's highest values for those who do not. It goes without saying in all this that the patient's individual convictions must always be respected.

The doctor and blame

It is not surprising in the field of cancer care, where cure is frequently impossible, that the anger which patients and their families naturally feel at the lack of success of their often very unpleasant treatment may be targeted at the doctor, whether justly or not.

This problem is usually avoided by ensuring that there is good communication with the ill person and their family. This involves spending time listening respectfully to them so that they feel their story has really been heard. Expressing their anger will also be cathartic and hence therapeutic.

Their anger may, of course, be justified, perhaps if there has been a delay in diagnosis or if they have been treated in a brusque and offhand manner; it is important in this situation to acknowledge the distress they feel.

The doctor may themselves feel anger at the patient; this can raise difficulties as there is rightly a taboo against a clinician venting their feelings on a sick and dying person. However, it is not necessary to like someone in order to give good medical care; it is usually possible to set aside temporarily such emotions and be objective in providing good care. The corollary of this is that the doctor must find someone outside the case to whom they can safely express their anger later on. On the rare occasions that the clinician finds they cannot maintain their objectivity, it is better to hand over care to another doctor.

THE INNER HEALER

It should be obvious by now that the person behind the various medical guises discussed is what makes these roles come alive and be effective in helping the dying. There is, so to speak, an inner healer who guides the practitioner in providing what the dying person most needs. The doctor can then move flexibly in and out of the various roles which are constructive and avoid those that are illusory and destructive. This requires a trust that there is within each carer an intuitive knowledge of the right approach to treating the dying. This is not to gainsay scientific knowledge; quite the opposite. There must be a working together – *caritas* and *scientia* – in harmony. There has been an unbalanced emphasis in Western medicine this century on the second part of this dyad, but there is now a welcome swing of the pendulum towards the first again and hospice medicine is playing its part in this happy rebirth.

REFERENCES

Coles, C.R. (1989) Diabetes education: theories of practice. *Practical Diabetes*, **6**, 119–202.

Hanks, P. (ed.) (1986) *The Collins English Dictionary*, 2nd edn, Collins, London.

Heyse-Moore, L.H. and Johnson-Bell, V.E. (1987) Can doctors accurately predict the life expectancy of patients with terminal cancer? *Palliative Medicine*, **1**, 165–6.

Ferrucci, P. (1982) *What We May Be*, Turnstone Press, Wellingborough.

Levine, S. (1987) *Healing into Life and Death*, Anchor Press, New York.

Saunders, C. and Sykes, N. (1993) *The Management of Terminal Malignant Disease*, 3rd edn, Edward Arnold, London, pp. 6–9.

Takeda, F. (1986) Results of field-testing in Japan of the WHO draft interim guideline on the relief of cancer pain. *The Pain Clinic*, **1**, 83–9.

Meeting social needs – the role of the social worker

8

The social work role and task in terminal illness and palliative care is varied, covering a range of duties, some more predictable than others and for which it is difficult to legislate in job descriptions. Over a number of years, working in both the voluntary and statutory sectors, my personal experience has reinforced the importance of being prepared for the unexpected – from advising on finances to arranging for a much-loved family pet to be rehoused, from negotiating with the Home Office on behalf of newly arrived political refugees to counselling people at major times of crises and despair. Whilst acknowledging the importance of life experience for those who are considering work in this field, it is also important to recognize the need for specialist skills and knowledge which, together with a flexible and pragmatic approach, will go some way to ensuring that the worker is, and is perceived as, a useful team member. Life experience and common sense are valuable assets and, together with a sound knowledge base of social, psychological and even political issues, will help to ensure that the social work contribution to the multidisciplinary team is a useful one.

Generally speaking, social work in a hospice setting can be described as a mix of practical and emotional help and advice. Frequently both aspects are closely interlinked and it should not be assumed that there is a clear division between them. Often the need to resolve pressing practical concerns can be a useful opening to discussion about the particular pressures that terminal illness can bring to people and their families and carers. It is difficult to concentrate on emotional reactions to diagnosis and prognosis of terminal illness if the most pressing immediate need is how to pay the electricity bill. A solution to that will often lead quite naturally to discussion and, hopefully, resolution in some way of deeper and more painful issues.

Practically, there is a variety of help available. The state welfare benefit system, although sometimes confusing to negotiate and apparently incomprehensible, does attempt to make reasonable provision for sick people, particularly those who are terminally ill. These benefits are administered by the Department of Social Security with devolved responsibility to local Benefit Agency offices. Different benefits are available, depending on whether one is under or over retirement age, and details of the most frequently used are given below.

Under retirement age

This is currently 60 for women and 65 for men.

Statutory Sick Pay/Sickness Benefit

National Insurance benefit, dependent on contributions, therefore claimant has to have been in work for relevant period. May lead to

Invalidity Benefit

In cases of long term sickness. To be replaced by Incapacity Benefit from April 1995.

Severe Disablement Allowance

Paid if ineligible for either of the above.

Income Support

Basic living allowance if no other financial means (and without savings between £3000–£8000). Can also claim for adult and child dependants.

Disability Living Allowance

Paid in two parts, attendance component and mobility component.

Attendance component
Special rules: for people with a terminal illness and a prognosis of six months or less. Confers eligibility at the higher rate and without the usual qualifying period of six months. Eligibility ceases after four weeks in hospital; there are different rules for longer term stays in voluntary hospices.

Mobility component
Paid at three different rates depending on severity of immobility (i.e. if unable to walk minimum (statutory) distance = high rate).

Over retirement age

Retirement pension

NI benefit paid at varying levels, dependent on NI contribution record. Reduces after six weeks in hospital, hospice or long term care. May be 'topped up' if below minimum current level with Income Support (see above).

Income Support (see above)

Attendance Allowance

Terminally ill people qualify under the Special Rules (see above). Stops after four weeks in hospital. Different rules for voluntary/independent hospitals and hospices.

Mobility component of DLA (see above)

Only claimable up to age 65 (or before 66th birthday if condition has been ongoing for at least six months previously). Payable for life. Not withdrawn if admitted to hospital, hospice or nursing home.

Industrial Injuries Benefit

For prescribed industrial diseases (such as mesethelioma following contact with asbestos). A claim has to be made by the person affected and the industrial link proven, which is a slow process. However, for many terminally ill people it is an option well worth pursuing since it may well provide additional financial security, both for the individual and a widowed spouse. The Society for Prevention of Asbestosis and Industrial Diseases (SPAID), a voluntary, self-help organization, can be useful in assisting this process.

Housing Benefit

A proportion of rent (both council and private) will be paid by the Housing Department of the Local Authority in appropriate cases. Claims are reassessed every six months. May continue after hospital/hospice admissions in certain cases.

Invalid Care Allowance

Payable to a carer of a sick or disabled person if working for 35+ hours each week and if the sick person receives either DLA or Attendance Allowance at either the middle or high rate. The carer must be aged 16–

65 and not earning more than £50 per week. It is taxed, but there are additional allowances for dependants (spouse and/or children).

Funeral payments

DSS will assist with funeral expenses in certain cases if the claimant (not the deceased person) receives either Income Support, Family Credit or Housing Benefit. There is no longer a statutory death grant and any estate left by the deceased person must go towards funeral expenses before any other financial claim on the estate can be allowed.

It is also possible in certain circumstances to get help with hospital fares, optical and dental charges and prescriptions. Generally, receipt of Income Support is the qualifying benefit, but it is important for individual claims to be made direct to the relevant Benefits Agency. There are other less frequently used allowances and it is always worth seeking advice, either from the local Benefits Agency (or the freephone line) or a Citizens Advice Bureau or similar organization offering welfare rights advice.

Other sources of funds for sick people are charities, both national and local. In particular, the Macmillan Fund is consistently generous with its funds, giving grants to people with cancer for immediate daily needs, such as heating and clothing, etc., but will also pay for special holidays or other particular needs which can be interpreted as improving the quality of life. The Sir Malcolm Sargent Cancer Fund helps with financial needs of families where there is an ill child, as does the Rowntree Trust.

There is a wide range of other practical issues which can be extremely important to people who are terminally ill. Making a will, an essentially practical procedure, can assist in coming to terms with what death and bereavement can mean to an individual and their family. It can be a way of aiding communication and indeed, opening up communication between people who are close to each other but finding it difficult to have open discussion about what is happening to them. Acknowledging the importance of making provision for one's dependants and making plans for the future can be an enabling and empowering process, albeit a painful one. The social worker has an important part to play in this process. By assisting with practical issues such as financial concerns, liaising with other agencies, negotiating plans for the future, jointly identifying areas of concern and tasks to be done, one is making an overt statement about the importance of the whole person in the context of the societal systems of which they are a part and attempting to make what is happening seem more manageable and bearable.

Dealing with important practical issues, particularly if there are young children involved and being able to ask for assistance in doing this, is an important beginning to the realization of the finality of death for one family member, but the expectation that life will continue for those remaining. There may be also special events which can be helpful, such as having a final holiday together. At its most simple this can leave happy memories and a more complex interpretation could point to the effects on mental and physical health in bereavement when careful joint planning has preceded it (Stroebe and Stroebe, 1987; Jewett, 1984).

WORKING WITH FAMILIES

Being sick, even slightly, can be a disabling experience, both physically and psychologically, with attendant feelings of loss of control and helplessness becoming paramount. This is particularly so in terminal illness. For example, change of role within the family can become a critical issue – the customary provider perhaps being unable to work and thus unable to provide materially or the main carer too ill to continue lifelong habits of looking after other family members. For everyone involved there will need to be major adjustments of many kinds – financial, social, emotional, etc.

With very few exceptions we are all members of some sort of societal grouping, families, extended family and relatives, friends, community groups, interest and self-help groups like schools and religious affiliations, many of which interact with each other in all sorts of ways throughout our lives. When thinking about our social groupings and in particular our closest groupings such as our families, I find a helpful simile is a mobile – a child's toy – a visual aid which gives a good example of how we all interact together. Touch one or more parts of the mobile and all the parts move. Touch one or more family member and the effects extend to everyone, not always predictably but movement and change are always there. Relate this to what is mentioned above, the need to take on different roles in times of crisis, to be aware of different needs within one's immediate group, and there is the beginning of coming to terms with a life crisis and the beginning of trying to make sense of what is happening, however unacceptable that may be.

When working with families facing the terminal illness of one of its members, the social worker has their own particular skills to bring. In my experience assessment of the current situation from a psychosocial perspective is the prime task. It is a means of gathering information and enabling the participants to make sense of it and make plans to deal with it. A useful tool here is the genogram or family tree. Completed together on an initial encounter, it fulfils several useful functions. It is an opportunity for introduction, acknowledges the need for partnership between health professional and patient, identifies family structure in a clear and comprehensive way, highlights relationships, strengths and weaknesses and can often clarify some of the 'rules' which operate and explain how earlier life events have been dealt with. Additions can be made easily and it can give an easily assimilated picture of events. Other relevant 'systems' can be readily included as appropriate (Burningham, 1986).

A family meeting can be mutually helpful. Potentially, it is an enabling, empowering process for the family; it shares information, acknowledges the importance of what is happening, gives permission for discussion and can go some way towards reducing feelings of helplessness. Hopefully, it will then be easier to identify tasks that need to be done, how they should be done and who should do them. It can also 'give permission' for tasks to be done. Groups need rules to survive and most of us are familiar with our own group or family rules. They may be simple rules associated with, for example, family chores – who does the washing up or the shopping. They may be more complex ones, like who is allowed to be openly angry. A central rule may be that one family member only makes all the major rules, which is fine until that person is no longer able to do so, at which stage new arrangements/rules need to be made to ensure a continuing 'fit' between family members. In this context, the loss of a family member is a major crisis which means that however relationships have operated in the past in this particular group, whether they have been good or bad, there will need to be major adjustments for the 'fit' between members to be satisfactory again.

LOSS, GRIEF AND BEREAVEMENT

Loss in its widest sense, in terms of separation from something or someone we are close to, is an experience we are all familiar with, although often we are less familiar with identifying its effects. It is, of course, part of our experience of daily living when applied to smaller material things, such as losing one's pen or one's purse, and part of our learning when dealing with more major life crises such as the loss of a faculty like sight, hearing or mobility or the death of someone, particularly someone who is well-known to us and well-loved by us.

Several writers, in particular Kübler-Ross (1970) and Parkes (1986), have identified stages of reaction to loss by bereavement and these findings can be readily applied to individuals who are experiencing personal loss in different ways. These stages are equally applicable to the loss of one's pen as to the loss of a person, albeit that the intensity of feeling and the pain are very different. Perhaps a major difference is that in smaller material losses, hope remains in some degree. The hope that it will one day turn up or be found unexpectedly somewhere remains, sometimes for a long time. In the context of loss of a person, this expectation is much more hopeless since the finality of death is irrevocable.

Kübler-Ross (1970) suggests a process of denial, anger, depression, bargaining and acceptance. If we apply this to a situation of our own – the lost pen – what happens?

- We look, disbelieving the evidence of our eyes – 'I'm sure it was here. I definitely remember. It *must* be here somewhere' (*denial*).
- Then, having searched, we often accuse those around us. 'It must have been moved. Why aren't my things left alone? (*anger*).
- 'If I could only find it, I would never forget where I put it down/be so careless, etc. again' (*bargaining*).
- 'It's really gone – no point in looking further. I shall have to buy another' (*acceptance*).

Obviously, this is a simple example, but the point I wish to make is that personal reactions to losses, both large and small, have areas of similarity. It is the degree of intensity of feeling which is different. Perhaps, also, the fact that another human being, another person, is involved is an essential crucial point. Marris (1992) clearly identifies this when talking about the experience of grief, how intertwined it is with human experience; it's not being widowed – the state of being which is so painful – it's being 'without'. Being without someone loved – being only a part instead of a whole – which is so awful and isolating.

Parkes (1986) identifies four stages of reaction:

1. Numbness and shock – disbelief at what has happened and anxiety at feelings of isolation and unreality from the world around one – a sometimes almost catatonic state of suspended animation, when immediate events are too frightening and horrific for reaction of any sort.
2. A period of acute grief, crying, even screaming, surges of emotion and often rage and anger.
3. A time of apathy and hopelessness, often of lassitude and inertia, where the whole business of living and continuing is completely overwhelming.
4. A time when the immediate and agonizing pain begins to subside and change and one learns to live in altered circumstances. The beginnings of making sense of something which seemed incomprehensible and wholly unacceptable.

In his work on grief, Worden (1983) suggests a similar spectrum of change: accepting the reality of the loss, experiencing the pain of grief, adjustment to the altered environment, transference and reinvestment of emotional energy.

It is important to remind ourselves that while all the above are wholly applicable theories, as human beings we are all very different in terms both of the depth of our reactions and the time and the ways in which we all deal with loss through bereavement and the concomitant grief. There is always a danger in applying theory over-rigidly in practice and it is not remotely helpful when counselling people in these circumstances to suggest that 'they should be over it by now' or that 12 months should be sufficient to arrive at stage 4 in the process. Or perhaps worst of all, that you know someone else who coped differently (i.e. better).

While considering aspects of loss, it is perhaps useful at this stage to acknowledge that it is a very different experience for the person who is ill than for their friends and relatives. For the sick person, it is an essentially individual and personal experience over which they have little final control. By the time someone arrives at a hospice, active treatment may well have finished or, as may be the case with younger people, may be used as a final attempt to slow down the progress of disease rather than as an attempt to cure.

Inherent in many of us is the need to protect those close to us. Frequently, on admission, as health professionals we are asked by relatives and families not to discuss prognosis or give information. It can be temptingly easy to collude with this, but I consider there is a place for professional integrity which cannot be justifiably ignored and I would fully endorse the policy (and practice) of honest, truthful answers to questions, while respecting individual values and beliefs, in all our dealings both professionally and privately. There is always, in my view, a kind of 'see-saw' operating between hope and realism, particularly in this area of work. In order to have a productive and useful working relationship with both the individuals and families we are working with and our team colleagues, I think it is essential that we are open and clear about what we are all, together, attempting to do.

One other aspect of working with people has not previously been mentioned here. To some extent, I have approached this chapter from an 'ideal' perspective with textbook stages of grief and planned family meetings. Although this can be the case, any discussion would be incomplete without acknowledgement of the fact that many relationships and much human interaction are decidedly less than ideal and, however carefully we plan in the light of our previous experience, there are few textbook situations where acceptance and change, or whatever other course of action has been decided upon, can be achieved. Add to that the differing perceptions and dynamics operative in any group, family or otherwise, and analysis and change within that group becomes increasingly complex. A longstanding poor marital relationship does not become loving and close overnight as a response to a diagnosis of terminal illness. Linked in with the feelings outlined above may be all sorts of other powerful emotions – relief, guilt and anger – that are insuppressible and hard to deal with either overtly or covertly. Being allowed to feel a range of emotions is an important part of grief work and therapy (Worden,

1983), but sometimes experiencing those emotions and acknowledging that they are there can be an overwhelming and frightening experience, as for example in the following:

> For many years, Jennie had cared for her elderly parents, having had to give up her career in her 40s when they became ill. Ten years later her father died. Five years after that, her mother was diagnosed as being terminally ill and after a protracted illness, during which time she was nursed at home by her daughter, becoming increasingly querulous and demanding, she finally died. Jennie, who prior to her mother's death openly admitted to being physically and emotionally drained, having never had a particularly good relationship with her mother, had gone on to discuss her feeling of relief and almost pleasurable anticipation at being free to make decisions for herself again after so long. It took many months of skilled counselling for Jennie to deal with a heavy burden of guilt for 'wishing her mother dead' before she was able to move on to the stage of transference and reinvestment for the future.

Chapter 20 develops further the many aspects of caring for bereaved people.

THE SOCIAL WORKER AS MULTIDISCIPLINARY TEAM MEMBER

Working in a multidisciplinary team can be an exciting, stimulating experience. It can be an opportunity to share skills and knowledge and develop a multifaceted approach to care by using the different attributes each team member can bring. However, good teamwork does not happen spontaneously. Organizational structures, clear policies and well-defined areas of acceptable practice throughout the respective disciplines are important as, without these, behaviour can become overcompetitive and destructive. Working in terminal care can be stressful and exhausting and without good management, effective support and supervision, it can be very lonely and isolated work.

Increasingly, particularly in hospice care, there is a blurring of professional boundaries and all team members will spend a part of their time counselling individuals and their families. Social workers frequently have a dual role in such teams and may on occasion be required to support other team members as well as patients. This seems to be an entirely valid use of social work time. Usually social workers are less involved in the initial clinical assessment but will be called in later when other issues have been identified. It is sometimes easier to talk to someone without direct clinical experience as the interchange can be less threatening and more equal.

A final point. This chapter would not be complete without acknowledging the necessity for all of us in this area of work sometimes simply to listen, without being overanalytical or too ready to assess, as concerns being told and retold can be valuable and helpful. To listen, perhaps many times to the same story, without judgement or impatience can create a safe environment, allowing change when the time is right.

REFERENCES

Burningham, J.B. (1986) *Family Therapy*, Routledge, London.

Kübler-Ross, E. (1970) *On Death and Dying*, Tavistock, London.

Marris, P. (1992) Grief, loss of meaning and society. *Bereavement Care*, **11**(2), 18–22.

Parkes, C.M. (1986) *Bereavement: Studies of Grief in Adult Life*, Penguin, Harmondsworth.

Stroebe, W. and Strobe, M.S. (1987) *Bereavement and Health*, Cambridge University Press, Cambridge.

Worden, J.W. (1983) *Grief Counselling and Grief Therapy*, Tavistock, London.

FURTHER READING

Disability Benefits Handbook (1993/94), Disability Alliance, London.

The value of physiotherapy 9

The modern hospice movement has revolutionized the care available to the terminally ill and their carers. Improved symptoms control has highlighted the place for rehabilitation in the care of the terminally ill. The role of the physiotherapist in the field of terminal care is a relatively new one but there is an increasing number of physiotherapists with a special interest in the particular needs of the terminally ill and the dying. The Association of Physiotherapists in Oncology and Palliative Care (ACPOPC, 1993) was recognized by the Chartered Society of Physiotherapists in 1990 and has a growing number of members nationwide.

The physiotherapist in a hospice setting works very much as a member of the multidisciplinary team, aiming to provide skilled and holistic care. The main focus of this care is the patient's quality of life. 'It is often possible to improve quality of life, regardless of prognosis, by helping an individual to achieve his maximum potential of functional ability and independence or to gain relief from distressing symptoms' (ACPOPC, 1993). The physiotherapist uses primarily physical means to this end but is concerned with the patient's psychological, emotional and spiritual comfort as well as their physical well-being.

Dame Cicely Saunders has commented that 'the way care is given can reach the most hidden place'. The way in which physiotherapy treatment is given to an individual who is terminally ill greatly influences its effect. Physical treatment, given with an awareness of and sensitivity to the whole individual, may have far-reaching effects which extend well beyond the presenting physical problem (Kearney, 1990).

Physiotherapeutic intervention within a hospice setting can be divided into the following categories:

1. pain control
2. restoration and maintenance of mobility
3. splinting
4. relief of respiratory symptoms
5. relaxation

6. reduction and control of limb oedema
7. treatment of clients with motor neurone disease (MND)
8. Treatment of clients with autoimmune deficiency syndrome (AIDS)
9. Teaching of lifting and handling skills.

PAIN CONTROL

The mainstay of pain control in a hospice setting is chemical. However, some particular forms of pain are responsive to the physical means of treatment available to the physiotherapist.

Pre-existing conditions presenting alongside malignant disease can be treated using the usual therapeutic agents, e.g. heat in its various forms, ice, ultrasound, interferential, laser and massage. Stiff, aching limbs and tense muscles may be eased by gentle passive or assisted active exercise (Judd, 1989). Uncomfortable spasticity caused by malignancy affecting the central nervous system may be eased by particular passive movements and advice on positioning.

Neuropathic pain is often responsive to transcutaneous electrical nerve stimulation (TENS). There are two different types of TENS: low TENS (low frequency, high intensity) may be used to relieve pain of central origin, e.g. thalamic pain and myofascial pains such as low back pain, torticollis and rheumatoid arthritis. Like acupuncture, low TENS is 'probably mediated by centrally released endogenous opioids' (Lundeberg, 1984). High TENS (high frequency, low intensity) is useful in relieving pain thought to have organic aetiology particularly neuropathic pain, e.g. where a cancer of the breast has invaded the cervical spine or bacterial plexus resulting in referred arm pain or where metastatic disease affecting the thoracic spine results in referred intercostal pain – 'the pain reducing effect of local spinal endogenous opioids (enkephalins)' (Lundeberg, 1984).

Some physiotherapists are also trained in the use of acupuncture and laser therapy for pain relief.

RESTORATION AND MAINTENANCE OF MOBILITY

Virtually all patients want to be able to walk! Mobility is frequently a key issue in how a patient perceives their quality of life. It is important for the physiotherapist to clearly identify the underlying cause of the immobility and so determine the efficacy of physiotherapy.

The physiotherapist needs to be honest with the patient and the family from the outset about what it is realistic to aim for. Realistic, short term goals need to be mutually agreed.

Mobilization of stiff joints and gentle strengthening exercises can be given as appropriate. Muscle fibrosis may occur following radiotherapy, necessitating stretching exercises to maintain ranges of movement. The preservation of joint mobility optimizes functional independence and makes nursing care easier. General debility in advanced disease contributes to weakness and the use of high dose steroids may result in a proximal 'steroid myopathy'. A programme of gentle exercise may be appropriate for patients with primary or metastatic brain disease resulting in motor and/or sensory loss. Rehabilitation may be appropriate according to the condition and prognosis of the patient.

> Pathological fractures and bony metastases may be managed conservatively or surgically, as appropriate. In the patient with a limited prognosis it is often appropriate to encourage early mobilization/ambulation within pain-free limits. Management may also include the assessment and provision of wheelchairs, transfer aids and adaptations.
>
> (ACPOPC, 1993)

A particular sensitivity on the part of the physiotherapist is required. A patient who is denying the reality of their illness may unconsciously attempt to draw the physiotherapist into colluding with them in this denial. A physiotherapist who is aware of and sensitive to these issues can be invaluable in supporting a patient who is slowly and painfully coming to terms with their illness and the consequent series of ongoing losses of independence. Relatives can be actively involved in treatment programmes and this can help to alleviate common feelings of helplessness. Involving relatives in passive movements, massage, etc. can also give permission to touch and be touched, providing a means of communication in which words are unnecessary.

SPLINTING

Appropriate simple splinting can add to a patient's comfort. A soft collar may support a weak and/or painful neck. Peripheral neuropathy may occur as a result of disease or chemotherapy and a splint may be used to support a paralysed hand or foot. Sub-Cuffs (a form of shoulder support) may be used to support a paralysed shoulder and prevent trauma to the capsule of the shoulder joint when the patient is being lifted. Corsets may be appropriate for patients with metastatic disease affecting the spine.

RELIEF OF RESPIRATORY SYMPTOMS

Dyspnoea, excessive secretions and ineffective coughs are common respiratory symptoms in patients with cancer, either as a direct result of disease in the lung or as a complication of malignancy elsewhere. The particular symptom and its cause needs to be isolated by the physiotherapist and the efficacy of physiotherapy determined, e.g. dyspnoea caused by gross ascites or a pleural effusion will not be relieved by physiotherapy and secretions distal to a large tumour are unlikely to be relieved by postural drainage. 'Pulmonary infection in neutropenic patients may require active but modified chest physiotherapy according to blood platelet levels' (ACPOPC, 1993).

Treatment can be given for pre-existing conditions such as chronic bronchitis, bronchiectasis or asthma but in the terminal phase of cancer the primary concern is the patient's comfort. Treatment techniques available to the physiotherapist to this end include positioning for postural drainage, breathing exercises, gentle vibrations and the use of humidifiers and nebulizers to aid expectoration. More aggressive forms of treatment are rarely tolerable or appropriate.

The use of low dose nebulized morphine to relieve dyspnoea in patients with advanced chronic lung disease has been studied and found to improve exercise endurance (Young, Daviskas and Keena, 1989). Research is currently being undertaken in the use of nebulized morphine to relieve dyspnoea in the terminally ill.

RELAXATION

The remit of the physiotherapist working in a hospice may include relaxation. For some patients, relentless anxiety and an inability to relax may become one of the main factors that impairs the quality of the living that they have left to do. It may result in a feeling of being isolated and get in the way of communication with the people close to them. The physiotherapist needs to spend time with the patient explaining clearly what a session of relaxation includes and exploring the nature of their anxieties. It is important that for further exploration of these anxieties with, for example, a counsellor or priest, the physiotherapist knows when to refer patients.

Care needs to be taken in preparing a quiet and warm environment. A simple sequence of relaxation may include muscle contraction/relaxation, breathing work and visualization. Music may also be appropriate.

Dr Michael Kearney, currently director of the Harold Cross Hospice in Dublin, describes how we as carers need to develop 'bifocal vision' to be able to truly address both the surface and deeper levels of an individual. He talks of the 'surface self' being 'visible, conscious and tangible' and the 'deeper self' as being 'invisible, unconscious and intangible'. A physiotherapist may develop and use this 'bifocal vision' when practising relaxation with patients to create an environment of safety in which an individual is able to open to a deeper level of themselves and so make use of the healing resources of the deeper self (Kearney, 1990).

Relaxation sessions may also be offered to groups of staff on a regular basis as part of a programme of supporting and taking care of the carers.

REDUCTION AND CONTROL OF LIMB OEDEMA

Lymphoedema may occur as a result of compression or internal occlusion of the lymphatics by tumour or as a result of surgical removal of and/or radiotherapy to the lymph nodes. Advice on the prevention of lymphoedema should be given to all patients at risk of developing lymphoedema. The management of lymphoedema may include some or all of the following.

1. Control of infection.
2. Massage
3. Sequential pressure pumps
4. Compression hosiery
5. Multilayered bandaging
6. Fluid mobilizing exercises
7. Health care advice.

Further information is available from the British Lymphology Interest Group, Administration Centre, Sir Michael Sobell House, Headington, Oxford OX3 7LJ (Badger and Twycross, 1988).

TREATMENT OF CLIENTS WITH MOTOR NEURONE DISEASE (MND)

Motor neurone disease is a progressive muscle wasting disease which results in a wide range of symptoms including altered muscle tone, muscle weakness, difficulty in walking, postural deformities, fatigue, dysarthria/disarturia and impaired vital capacity. The physiotherapist may use active and passive exercise, stretching, positioning and splints to maintain regular exercise programmes to optimize remaining muscle power. Exercise programmes need to be frequently monitored and reviewed according to the changing condition of the patient. Callipers, walking aids and wheelchairs may be provided to maintain and optimize functional ability and independence. Active chest physiotherapy may be appropriate in the preterminal phase of the disease.

More information about MND and the support and equipment available to those who have the disease can be obtained from the Motor

Neurone Disease Association, P.O. Box 246, Northampton NN1 2PR (ACPOPC, 1993).

TREATMENT OF CLIENTS WITH AUTOIMMUNE DEFICIENCY SYNDROME (AIDS)

The wide range of symptoms which may occur as a result of the human immunodeficiency virus (HIV), e.g. lung infections, cerebral lesions, peripheral neuropathies and arthritis, mean that the physiotherapist may be called upon to use a wide variety of treatment techniques. Intervention may include management of respiratory difficulties, using modified Bobath and other rehabilitation approaches when appropriate and supplying splints, walking aids and wheelchairs (ACPOPC, 1993).

TEACHING OF LIFTING AND HANDLING SKILLS

The Health and Safety at Work Act of 1974 stressed the importance of safe lifting and handling. The European Commission legislation of 1993 made it a legal obligation for employers to provide education in spinal awareness and safe lifting and handling techniques and to provide the necessary equipment. Physiotherapists working in hospices, as in other areas or work, are actively involved in assessing tasks that require lifting and manual handling and in teaching other members of the multidisciplinary team skilled and safe lifting strategies and techniques.

In conclusion, the role of the physiotherapist in the care of the terminally ill is a very varied and fulfilling one. As for other members of the multidisciplinary team, as well as their professional skills and knowledge the physiotherapist brings a personal element. Perhaps it is partly the recognition of this by those working with the terminally ill that draws an increasing number of physiotherapists to this special and rewarding field of caring.

REFERENCES

Association of Chartered Physiotherapists in Oncology and Palliative Care (ACPOPC) (1993) *Physiotherapy in Oncology and Palliative Care. Guidelines for Good Practice*, Chartered Society of Physiotherapy, 14 Bedford Row, London.

Badger, C. and Twycross, R. (1988) *Management of Lymphoedema*, Sir Michael Sobell House, Churchill Hospice, Oxford.

Judd, M. (1989) Physiotherapy and the dying patient, in *Caring for the Dying Patient and the Family*, 2nd edn, (ed. J. Robbins), Chapman & Hall, London, pp. 133–7.

Kearney, M. (1990) Spiritual pain. *The Way*, **1**, 47–54.

Lundeberg, M.D. (1984) Electrical stimulation for the relief of pain. *Physiotherapy*, **70**(3), 88–100.

Young, I.H., Daviskas, E. and Keena, V.A. (1989) Effect of low dose nebulised morphine on exercise endurance in patients with chronic lung disease. *Thorax*, **44**, 387–90.

FURTHER READING

Frampton. V.M. (1982) Pain control with the aid of transcutaneous nerve stimulation. *Physiotherapy*, **68**(3), 77–81.

Gray, R.C. (1989) The role of physiotherapy in hospice care. *Physiotherapy Practice*, **5**, 9–16.

10 Care of the dying child and the family

The child is not a small adult and this concept is especially true when caring for the dying child. The nurse has to recognize children's different levels of understanding according to their individual ages and experiences, to be able to talk to the child about death and dying in a meaningful way and to be able to identify their physical and psychological needs. They need to have knowledge of how children respond to illness and how to plan and implement specific care to meet these needs.

Family centred care is now the focus of paediatric nursing so the paediatric nurse also has to act as an educator and support to help parents care for their child. They have to be able to appreciate and respond to the varied emotions displayed by parents whose child is dying. They need to be able to recognize the psychological impact on the affected child's healthy siblings and help them to cope with this traumatic situation.

Last, but not least, the nurse needs to be able to be aware of their own values and beliefs concerning death and to have a strategy for releasing their own emotions.

The aim of this chapter is to provide nurses involved with caring for the dying child with some guidelines for dealing with these issues. Firstly the child's understanding of death is considered, followed by suggestions for communicating with dying children and supporting parents. Some of the common physical problems of dying children are explained together with strategies for symptom relief. The issue of involving parents in care is explored and also the advantages and disadvantages of nursing the child at home. Also, the effect of terminal care upon the nurse is discussed. Finally, the areas of miscarriage, stillbirth and neonatal death are covered.

CHILDREN'S PERCEPTION OF DEATH

Most children have some ideas about death. Their games often involve death, usually in a violent way, probably as the result of television and cartoons. Some children have also had some experience of the reality of death because of the death of a grandparent or family pet. The ideas about death will be different for every child because of their individual experience but also according to their stage of cognitive development.

The work of Piaget (1954) demonstrates that children's understanding varies between different age groups and that this variation is largely predictable. Several researchers have found that these developmental changes can also be seen in children's understanding of illness. Children's understanding of death has not been studied so extensively, possibly because it is a more difficult topic to explore with young children, but the few studies which are available indicate that this understanding is also linked to age.

These studies relate to children over the age of two years. It is difficult to know whether children under this age have any awareness or understanding of death. Preschool children (2–5 years) are described by Piaget (1954) as being at a preoperational (or prelogical stage). During this stage children do not think logically and tend to view ideas only from their own perspective. At this age they are unable to accept the irreversibility of death and can only relate it to their understanding of sleep which is a temporary process. This may be partly due to the influence of cartoon characters who are always revived after violent occurrences. They conceive the dead person as existing somewhere else (e.g. in heaven or under the ground). Often death is associated with darkness which may be connected with the child's experience of sleep which mostly occurs at night, in the dark. Vidovich (1980) reports that a five year old child who was dying was heard to ask: 'When will it be dark? Will mummy be here when it gets dark?'.

The egocentricity of young children may cause them to feel responsible in some way for the death of a loved one because they have been naughty. These feelings may be perpetuated if they find themselves neglected because the rest of the family are overcome by grief. They also find it difficult to perceive death as a normal event which happens to everyone including themselves.

Children between the ages of five and eight are beginning to understand that death is a natural event. Lansdown and Benjamin (1988) found that 60% of children in this age group had realistic ideas about the finality of death although they were still largely unaware that it could happen to them during childhood. Although this reasoning is more sophisticated than that of the younger child, the cause of death is still generally seen as external and there may still be concerns about death being infectious, occurring at a certain age or after a specific event. It is also difficult for children at this age to perceive the future and therefore they do not have the ability to recognize gradual deterioration in themselves or others or to consider what may follow this deterioration.

During middle childhood, children acquire an even more realistic picture of death and recognize it as an inevitable and universal process. They are also able to gather information together and begin to make reasoned judgements about that information. Thus, children who are terminally ill can come to realize that death is imminent.

Piaget terms adolescence 'that formal operational stage of cognitive development'. This is the age at which children can think beyond the present and conceptualize the future. They can imagine processes such as death, even if they have not directly experienced such events. They can also appreciate that emotions can affect body functions. Because the adolescent is able to visualize the future and has goals and aspirations for adulthood, they may express anger and resentment that death has interfered with these.

COMMUNICATION AND THE DYING CHILD

Piaget's stages of cognitive development is a useful guide when caring for dying children but the nurse also needs to consider the individual child. Reilly *et al.* (1983) discovered that children who had personal experience of death generally had an accelerated understanding of death. It is therefore important that the nurse knows as much about the child as an individual as possible so that they can communicate at an appropriate level. This understanding of the child as an individual will also help them to become aware of the child's willingness, or otherwise, to talk about dying.

Bluebond-Langer (1989) suggests that children often appreciate the seriousness of their illness even when they have not been informed of their condition. They often choose not to discuss their fears of dying because they have learnt that death is not something that is talked about openly.

Lansdown (1980) summarizes the stages that children pass through when recognizing the inevitability of their own death:

'I am very sick'
'I have an illness which can kill people'
'I have an illness which can kill children'
'I may not get better'
'I am dying'

Thus the pretence that the child is not fatally ill and an unwillingness to pursue difficult questions about the nature of dying is an affront to children's intelligence. A tendency to avoid the issue may lead to the child losing trust in the nurse.

One of the priorities for paediatric nurses is to obtain children's trust. Trust can only be gained through honest and accurate information. Nurses working with dying children should be aware of their feelings, be truthful and take time to listen (Jolly, 1981). Nurses often want detailed prescriptive advice on talking to dying children which may reflect their own fear of confronting strong emotions and personal difficulties in coming to terms with death. Wright (1991) suggests that it is essential for nurses to explore their own feelings about death before they can openly discuss dying with others. As Lansdown (1980) states, 'The more we know, the less we fear and the more we can see through to the normal bits of the person underneath'.

Every communication with a dying child will be different. It is impossible to determine strategy in advance of the situation because responses will be determined by the individual child's questions. A useful guide for communicating with the dying child is given by Judd (1993) who suggests that the nurse's role is to listen rather than to inform, to avoid lying and to be led by the child about how much to say at any moment. Cues can be taken from the child's non-verbal communication as well as from their actual words. The listener should respond to the feelings expressed, simply and without embarrassment, which will help the child to feel safe to continue the conversation. It is important to allow the child to direct the pace of the exchange and to admit uncertainty rather than to try and answer unanswerable questions. It is more important for the child to have someone with whom to share their feelings than to have to decipher complicated answers.

As with adults, it is useful to ask why the question is being asked. Swaffield (1985) describes a nine year old who asked if he was dying because he had a headache as his mother always said she was dying when she had a bad headache.

Although the child has a **right** to know if he is dying, he may not have the **need** to know. Lansdown (1980) supports this idea that not every child should know everything. Continuity of care should enable the nurse to build up a close relationship with the child so that they can recognize when the child has the need to communicate and so that they feel safe enough to raise their questions. Children will interact in this way provided they are cared for in a warm, loving, supportive and safe environment (Vidovich, 1980).

SUPPORT FOR THE FAMILY

Paediatric nursing is concerned with supporting the family as much as it is about caring for the child. This is particularly pertinent when caring for the dying child. Studies as well as personal accounts have shown that this support is often lacking for parents whose children have died (Bennett, 1984). Davies (1979) voices parents' reactions very succinctly when she describes her feelings when her daughter Sarah was dying: 'You feel totally inadequate, lost, hopeless, stupid'.

Other emotions experienced by parents caring for a dying child are shock, confusion, fear, anger and guilt. Parents are often so shocked on being told that their child is dying, even if this is confirmation of their own suspicions, that they do not hear any further explanation. The nurse needs to give parents time to come to terms with this news and then provide opportunities to answer questions. Following this initial shock, parents then feel confused about their parental role. They no longer feel able to care for their child and they do not know how to divide their time between the dying child and the other members of the family. Their lives have been completely altered by this event and they do not know how to cope. Mothers particularly experience a loss of control or mastery perhaps because they often bear the burden of the caring role (Jennings, 1992). The nurse can help the parents to rediscover their role, involve them in the care of their child and support them in making decisions about sharing their time and presence amongst other family members. Muller *et al.* (1992) suggest that this is best achieved by a primary nurse who can get to know the family's values, beliefs and relationships.

Confusion can also be due to fear. Many parents are frightened of the actual death and often visualize that this will be violent and painful for the child. They are also frightened that they will not be able to cope with the child's physical care or be able to control their emotions. Like nurses, they often have difficulty in communicating with their child about dying and they sometimes dread the questions that the child might ask because they fear that they will be unable to respond. The nurse needs to be able to give the parents time and opportunity to express these fears and provide them with simple guidelines on how to deal with the child's questions.

Anger may arise from this fear and confusion, often as an expression of despair. The fight to understand the situation and control the emotions produces anger which may be directed at the nurse. It is not easy for the nurse to accept such emotions but as Wright (1991) acknowledges, the verbal expression of anger can often aid catharsis. If the nurse can accept this and remain supportive, they can strengthen their relationship with the family.

Often an angry outburst will then cause parents to feel guilty at causing distress to others. Guilt is a common reaction amongst parents of dying children. They may feel guilty because they failed to recognize and respond effectively to the symptoms of the child's illness; because the illness is hereditary; or they believe because their behaviour (e.g. smoking) somehow triggered the illness. The nurse should be alert to parental expressions of guilt or self-blame and assist parents to examine the validity of their apportionment of responsibility. If necessary, this may also involve helping them to forgive themselves or others.

These emotional reactions to the dying child are not confined to the parents. Bluebond-Langer (1989) recognizes that the destructive effects of terminal illnesses involve the whole family. In particular, siblings of the dying child may feel rejected and neglected as the sick child becomes the centre of attention (Collinge and Stewart, 1983). Healthy siblings may feel anxiety about their own health (Cairns *et al.*, 1979).

Jealousy and resentment may result from parental preoccupation with the dying child. This, in turn, may lead to feelings of guilt, as the siblings try to direct attention upon themselves (Burton, 1975). If these effects are not recognized and/or managed, behavioural problems such as enuresis, school phobia, depression and abdominal pain may ensue. The nurse can help parents to recognize the needs of siblings and by being with the dying child, can enable them to spend time alone with their other children. The nurse can also help the parents to meet siblings' needs by accepting their involvement in the care of the sick child (Doyle, 1987). The parents may also need to maintain as normal a family routine, including discipline, as possible for all members of the family. This helps the affected child and the siblings to feel secure (Cairns *et al.*, 1979).

Such enormous responsibilities for parents in these situations may cause break-up of the family (Gonda and Ruark, 1984). Hill (1993) also recognizes that the strain of a child's terminal illness upon a marital relationship can be destructive. The stress involved in coming to terms with the varied emotions described above combined with the sheer physical exhaustion caused by trying to maintain normal work and family routines whilst caring for the dying child may often cause conflict. The nurse should be aware of these potential tensions and as far as possible, try to help parents to spend time together and also give them time to express feelings separately and together. Muller *et al.* (1992) suggest that the use of outside agencies such as social workers or CRUSE may be helpful. Jennings (1992) suggests that mothers find it easier than fathers to express and work through their feelings. Nurses need to be alert to the possibility that this may be because mothers are more available or that female emotions are easier for nurses to deal with. Consequently, it may be that fathers are given less opportunity to share their feelings especially if these are hidden as they strive to demonstrate strength.

MEETING PHYSICAL NEEDS

Relief of pain

Pain is the most common symptom in dying patients and the aspect which is most feared by the child and their parents. Eighty percent of dying children will experience pain (Hill, 1993). If it is not managed well it can lower morale and ability to cope.

The first stage in relieving the dying child's pain is an accurate assessment of the severity, the type and the cause of the pain. Assessment of pain in children is often complicated by the child's inability to express themselves clearly. This may be due to a lack of vocabulary in the infant or child with special needs, because the child is unwilling to distress their parents or because they are frightened that pain relief will be given via an injection.

Observing physiological changes can be a useful assessment of pain in infants who are less influenced by fear and stress. With toddlers, it is useful to listen to comments from parents who know their child well enough to recognize changes in behaviour which may indicate pain. In this way, the nurse can begin to recognize the subtle changes in a child which reveal their individual response to pain.

Objective ways of assessing pain using the child's own viewpoint are invaluable in planning and evaluating pain relief. Although still not used widely in the management of paediatric pain, assessment tools can be used successfully in children as young as three years. Beyer (1984) developed the 'oucher' scale for young children who are asked to choose one face from six expressive pictures which most closely reflects their feelings about their pain.

Between the ages of four and seven the poker chip method of assessment can be used. The child is given four poker chips and asked to indicate the number of chips which best corresponds with their pain. Thus they select one chip if the pain is slight, but four chips if they find the pain unbearable (Alder, 1990).

Once children can identify colours the Eland colour tool can be used. The child is asked to select several colours to represent degrees of pain and may help the nurse to colour in the assessment chart accordingly. At each assessment of pain they are then asked to choose the colour which best reflects their current pain.

Children over the age of seven can usually use an adult visual analogue scale to indicate the severity of their pain and may also be able to describe the type of pain more accurately than the younger child whose vocabulary and understanding is limited.

Identification of the type of pain may help the nurse to establish the cause of the pain and consequently to respond to it in the most appropriate way. In younger children this information may be aided by knowing the site of the pain. Ekland and Anderson (1977) showed that 97% of children aged 4–10 years can correctly identify the site of pain on a body outline.

The planning and implementation of pain relief should follow established models unless the child presents in severe pain. There should be a gradual progression from a non-opioid analgesia to a weak opioid and finally a strong opioid (Hill, 1993). In her moving account of the care of a dying teenager, Hunt (1990) describes the gradual progression from 30 mg dihydrocodeine daily to 330 mg twice daily of morphine slow-release tablets in the successful management of terminal pain. Unfortunately, there are still many myths about the use of opioids for children and the nurse may have to act as the patient's advocate to ensure that the dying child receives the appropriate analgesia at the correct strength for their pain. If this is not achieved the child will experience the negative effects of insufficient or overpowerful analgesia which will only cause them and their parents further distress.

Pain in terminal illness is usually constant and for this reason analgesia should be given regularly so that the child can maintain a continuous level of pain relief. To ensure this goal is met the adequacy of the relief should be reassessed regularly. Oral analgesia is the route of choice for children but is not necessarily accepted by all children. The nurse may need to be imaginative in the use of play to ensure the child accepts medicine on a regular basis. When nausea and vomiting do not allow oral medication, subcutaneous analgesia can be given using a syringe pump. This method has the advantage of enabling the child to remain mobile. Hill (1993) suggests that pain-free mobility should be one of the goals for pain relief. She suggests that the primary goal is to enable relief from pain during sleep. Secondly, the nurse should aim to provide sufficient analgesia to give the child complete relief from pain at rest and finally the child should be able to move around without pain.

Psychological methods of pain relief may also provide a useful adjunct to medication. Hypnosis, distraction techniques and the use of imagery and relaxation can all be helpful in the management of children's pain (Alder, 1990). They are relatively easy for children of all ages to use and have the advantage of giving them some control over their situation. The nurse should not forget the influence of fear upon pain and aim to keep the child as relaxed as possible with explanations of treatment and reassurance. Simple measures such as touch, being settled into a more comfortable position or the presence of a nurse or parent for a frightened child may help to relax the child and reduce the intensity of the pain.

Nausea and vomiting

Nausea and vomiting are common problems for children who are dying and can cause them much distress. The commonest causes are constipation, raised intracranial pressure or excessive pharyngeal secretions (Hill, 1993). Prescribed antiemetics should act on the site of the cause. When the cause is uncertain, a combination of antiemetics which act on different sites may be useful. When oral medication cannot be used, antiemetics can be given rectally or via a subcutaneous infusion.

Nausea and vomiting are sometimes seen as a side effect of opioids but are usually only troublesome initially. Hill (1993) estimates that 25–30% of children will experience problems when opioids are first used but generally overcome these in 5–10 days. She does not recommend the regular use of prophylactic antiemetics and suggests haloperidol (25–50 μg/kg) or cyclizine (up to 75 mg daily) only if vomiting occurs.

Anorexia

Pain and/or nausea and vomiting may cause anorexia which is often more of a problem for parents than the child. The child may be helped by small frequent snacks of favourite foods rather than two or three large meals a day. Parents may be reassured by understanding that the child's energy requirements are less because of their relative immobility. They may also feel that they are able to help the problem by supplying the child with small portions of favourite foods.

Dyspnoea

Dyspnoea in the dying child may be caused by secondary lung tumours, pleural effusions or direct respiratory centre invasion in children with malignant disease. It may be due to the primary disease process, as in cystic fibrosis, or to respiratory muscle dysfunction in children with degenerative disease. Often a chest infection will exacerbate the primary cause.

Treatment of dyspnoea is often empirical. Dyspnoea is frightening for the child and the parents and their anxiety can often aggravate the problem. The nurse can do much simply by providing a reassuring and calm atmosphere. Careful positioning of the child using a bean bag or elevating the head of the bed may increase their comfort. A frightened child can be helped by being supported in an upright position on a parent's or nurse's lap.

Excess secretions may be overcome by gentle physiotherapy or the administration of hyoscine. A dry cough which prevents rest and sleep can be helped with simple linctus which is usually well accepted by children and will act as a suppressant.

Constipation

Constipation is an inevitable consequence of opioid use and children who are prescribed strong opioids should also be given regular prophylactic laxatives. Constipation leads to discomfort, nausea, vomiting and anorexia and causes needless distress to the child and their parents.

Danthron (12.5–25 mg) is well accepted by children and can be given once at bedtime, but it acts by increasing gut mobility and can cause abdominal cramps. It is not useful for children in nappies or those who have become incontinent as prolonged faecal contact with the skin can cause irritation and excoriation.

Lactulose (10–25 ml) acts by osmosis and softens stools by maintaining a volume of fluid in the bowel. It is a useful laxative when given regularly but children often dislike its taste and a twice daily dose is recommended.

The nurse should be aware of the child's usual bowel habits and be alert to any changes in these so that the discomfort and distress of constipation do not occur.

Anxiety

If the anxiety of the dying child and their family is not managed it will aggravate the physical symptoms. Rodin (1983) has clearly shown that the anxiety of a child is clearly related to the anxiety of their parents. Harris' (1981) study showed that just having a child in hospital caused parents to become uncertain and frightened. It is easy to imagine how these feelings are magnified if the child has a terminal illness. Parental anxiety is reduced by having information about their child's treatment and the hospital routine and being able to discuss their future (Sadler, 1988). They may also be helped by reassurance that their feelings are neither unusual or silly (Muller *et al.*, 1992).

Although helping parents with their anxieties will also help to calm the child, the nurse should also give the child time to express their feelings. They will need reassurance about new and unfamiliar symptoms and information about how these can be managed. Play can be useful both to enable the child to express their feelings but also to act as a diversion and to continue the child's normal routine.

Anxiety can cause insomnia. In some situations children are so frightened of not waking that sleep is impossible. It is important to enable the child to discuss such fears but it may be necessary to give a small dose of an anxiolytic, such as lorazepam, at bedtime which will not cause daytime sedation.

Depression

Often increasing physical deterioration in the child who is dying causes depression. This is often manifest as a psychological regression with the child becoming very dependent and clinging to one parent. It may also cause a withdrawal and loss of interest in normal activities such as play or watching television.

The nurse can help the child by encouraging them to express their feelings. Such expression of feelings may be initiated by the nurse's acknowledgement of them; 'I know you are feeling sad' or 'This must be very hard for you' may be useful ways to open the discussion (Judd, 1993).

The nurse may also help by enabling the child to achieve control over their daily routine. The dying child often feels that they have no control over events which sometimes increases their despair and dependence on others. They can be encouraged to make decisions about their care and their efforts towards independent behaviour should be encouraged.

INVOLVING PARENTS IN CARE

Casey (1988) has described paediatric nursing as being a partnership with parents. It has been strongly suggested since 1947 that parents be involved in their child's care (Spence, 1947). Parents know their child best and can provide continuity of care and security. Consolvo (1986) found that mothers showed significantly less anxiety when they were able to be involved in their child's care. Siblings may also be helped by being involved in care. They can play with the ill child or help in practical care such as making drinks. Cleary *et al.* (1986) discovered that the child cared for by their family cried less and spent less time alone than children who were nursed unaccompanied.

Parents are willing and able to participate in their child's care and often are keen to be involved more than nurses believe they are (Webb, Hull and Madeley, 1985). But they cannot be expected to do so alone. The Audit Commission (1993) reported that often parents' perception of the reason for their involvement in care was because the nurses were too busy. Casey's (1988) notion of partnership and negotiated care with parents was not always apparent to parents.

When they have a child who is dying parents may feel they are losing control and they may see the nurse as taking over that control. A supportive relationship with the parents should enable the nurse to help them maintain their role as decision makers and carers. All care should be negotiated and the nurse's and parents' roles clearly defined. At the same time the nurse should be alert to parental needs, abilities and stresses. Parental involvement can range from a presence at the bedside to total care of the child with supervision from the nurse (Evans, 1977).

Parents may need support from the nurse to take time away from the dying child and not to feel guilty about the need for sleep, relaxation or time at home or work.

To provide the parents with both physical and psychological support the nurse needs to be available to answer questions, explain care and to listen and respond to spoken and unspoken fears, anxieties, stresses and strains.

HOME OR HOSPITAL CARE?

Goldman *et al.* (1990) consider that almost all children prefer to die at home in familiar surroundings. Caring for the dying child at home seems to reduce the long term problems of depression and guilt experienced by bereaved parents and siblings (Lauer *et al.*, 1983). However, Bluebond-Langer (1989) disputes this and suggests that siblings often feel confused, rejected and lonely when their home environment changes to care for the dying child. To ensure a positive outcome parents caring for dying children at home need the support of the paediatric nurse.

If the child has been in hospital, parents need clear instructions and advice. It has been shown that this is not always forthcoming. MacDonald (1988) studied the discharge information given to mothers and found that many left hospital with unclear or insufficient explanations. Muller *et al.* (1992) believe that the success of home care depends on the availability of community paediatric teams who can provide 24-hour support. Goldman *et al.* (1990) describe the success of providing such a 24-hour 'on call' system. In spite of continuing support for the Platt report (1959) recommendations to establish specialist nursing teams of this type for the home care of children, paediatric community nursing teams are few. In 1989 Whitting (1990) found that only 12.6% of district health authorities employed such teams with some teams consisting of only one registered paediatric nurse.

It must also be recognized that not all parents will feel able physically or psychologically to care for their dying child at home. These parents should not be made to feel guilty at such a decision. Harris (1981) found that care at home sometimes fails because of lack of family resources and/or community support. The decision to care for a dying child at home needs careful assessment of all the factors involved in negotiation with the parents, siblings and affected child. Provision should be made for alternatives if home care does fail so parents recognize that they can return to hospital care without needing to feel inadequate.

An alternative to home and hospital care is the hospice which will centre care entirely around the support of the family (Copsey, 1981). The nurse may be the person to discuss with the family the best option for them and their child.

CARE OF THE NURSE

Caring for dying children is stressful. Vidovich (1980) found that the death of a child may cause the nurse to feel failure, guilt, anger or overwhelming sadness. Support for nurses caring for the dying child and their family is essential if burnout is to be avoided. Siedel (1981) suggests that a systematic approach to death education in nurse training may partly help to prepare nurses for meeting the needs of the dying. She also proposes that such a programme allows nurses to come to terms with their own beliefs about dying so that they are better to cope with their own emotional needs.

Muller *et al.* (1992) suggest that regular support group meetings be held for nurses caring for dying children. This gives these staff the opportunity to acknowledge and discuss actions such as symptom control and talking with parents. Saunders (1982) suggests that for many nurses a support group provides encouragement that they are doing the right thing.

Nurses need to be informed of a child's death even when they have been off duty. They need to know what happened in order to cope with their own feelings and support the other children on the ward. Many nurses also find it useful to be given time to attend the child's funeral to allow them to say their final goodbye.

MISCARRIAGE, STILLBIRTH AND NEONATAL DEATH

Death before life has been established is divided into miscarriage, stillbirth and neonatal death and can mean the end of hopes, dreams and plans and immediate parenting for the woman and her partner.

The grief that follows in any of the circumstances is intensely personal, a private agony, often too painful to share. Acceptance of what has happened, for whatever reason, is the final stage in the grieving process. Saying goodbye is an important act of acceptance, but the context of the farewell often makes it a difficult goal to achieve for the mother, her partner and family.

The health professionals who are caring for the parents when death of the baby occurs also suffer. The most frequent question asked by both parents and professionals is 'Why did this happen?', 'What did I do wrong?'. Education and support for professionals is essential in order to enable them to support and care for the parents.

It is not necessary for the professional to have experienced a similar personal tragedy for them to be able to help and share the emotions and feelings of the bereaved parents. However, the development of a caring, sympathetic, empathetic attitude is essential. Being able to listen, to say sorry, to be honest and open with the parents will aid the development of the grieving process and create good memories of what is essentially a very confusing and sad time.

Kohner and Henley (1991) offer many moving accounts from parents who have suffered miscarriage, stillbirth and neonatal death. They point out that for each parent, the death of their baby has a very particular meaning and has little to do with the timing of the loss.

Miscarriage

Miscarriage occurs when the baby dies before 24 weeks gestation. Many parents who suffer a miscarriage find that their loss is regarded by professionals as a lesser event than a stillbirth and is often therefore perceived by professionals as less upsetting (Kohner and Henley, 1991).

Once a pregnancy has been confirmed and even before this for many women, a bond has been formed with the baby evolving within the uterus. The establishment of the pregnancy begins for some parents before the baby is conceived. Jolly (1989) suggests stages of bonding as shown in Figure 10.1.

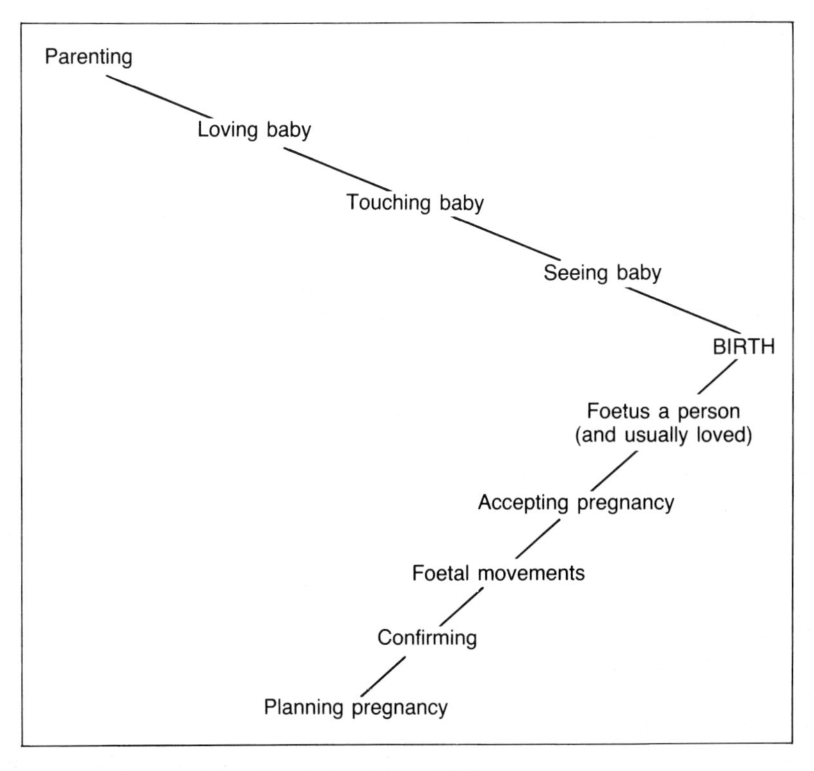

Figure 10.1 Stages of bonding (after Jolly, 1989).

It is important to remember that some pregnancies are unplanned and some are complicated by lack of partner, social and economic deprivation, infertility, previous death of a baby and physical or psychological problems. All these factors can affect the grieving process if death of the baby occurs.

When a baby dies whilst in the uterus, before 24 weeks gestation, medical terminology may describe the baby as an unviable fetus. We should remember that to the parents the baby is a baby from the moment of conception. When miscarriage occurs, it is often glossed over by the attending staff, almost as if it had not occurred at all. One woman described her feelings towards staff in this way:

> The doctors want to 'scrape' you clean as quickly as possible to get rid of what they call 'the retained products of conception' but do not seem to realize that a mother cannot forget quite so easily. It is insensitive – it was my baby that they were talking about.

On the other hand, a parent with a very positive experience of hospital care said:

> When they said I would lose the baby, they (the staff) did everything they could have possibly done to help me. They listened to me, they gave me mementoes of the birth, a footprint, a handprint, a photograph. She was so very tiny but I loved her; this helped me so much in the months that followed.

Partners and family are often at a loss as to the best way of helping. There is a real need for more recognition by society and all carers that the woman perceived this as her baby no matter what the stage of gestation before birth. She had hopes and fears, aspirations for the child's future and the parents will have made preparations in the home in readiness to receive the child after the birth.

Women, their partners and relatives often wish to see the dead baby and every effort to accommodate this wish should be made. The carers are privileged participants in the event of a miscarriage and it is their attitude, their actions and words which will influence the parents as to whether they see the dead baby after delivery. Encouraging words which describe the perfection of feet and hands and other parts of the child take away the fear which may be present in the parents and actively encourage them to look at and see their dead baby. Both the seeing and the touching introduces reality to the process and engenders the commencement of the grieving process.

Burial is a difficult subject, as before 24 weeks gestation there is no official recognition of viability. Parents may take the dead baby home and some parents do this and then arrange the preferred ceremony, religious or otherwise and the burial of the body.

Today hospitals are much more sensitive to this issue, some having created memorial gardens where flowers can be planted. All most certainly arrange for photographs of the baby. Often the baby is laid in a small basket, dressed in normal clothing. These examples give realism to the death of the baby: 'It really did happen, I was pregnant, I did have a baby'. These are important factors for the mother's mental health and a healthy approach to any future pregnancy.

For each parent the death of their baby has a particular meaning and has little to do with the timing of the death. Hospitals are now realizing that women and their partners need special help at this time. Bereavement counsellors, nurses and midwives and individuals with special training are assisting women and helping them to make the death of their baby a reality.

Termination of pregnancy for abnormality

When antenatal diagnostic examinations such as ultrasound scanning or blood tests confirm that abnormality of the fetus exists this is a particularly difficult and trying time for parents. They need to make a decision as to whether the pregnancy is to be terminated based on the information they have been given. They need to talk through the situation in privacy and as often as they need, to be able to come to an agreed joint decision. The parents will require sympathetic and informed support on the options open to them. What will happen if they decide to have the pregnancy terminated? Will pain relief be available? Will they be able to see the baby? These are some of the common fears. They need to be reassured that they will be supported throughout the labour and the birth, preferably by the same midwife.

Support After Termination For Abnormality (SATFA) is an organization which can help both the professional and the parent.

Termination of pregnancy for other reasons

When a woman chooses to terminate her pregnancy for other reasons it is often regarded and referred to as 'her own fault'. The aftermath of guilt and the repression of feelings can often cause depression. McAll (1982) states that women are often haunted by the cries of their dead child and that, far from putting the matter out of their minds, many women have secretly given their babies names and many feel that they have been instrumental in committing murder.

Carers are professionals and no matter what decision the woman has taken, she should be supported and cared for and not classified as irresponsible. It is so very easy to help parents create memories and enhance positive feelings. A kind word, recognition and empathizing with the emotions and feelings go a long way to help parents come to terms with the death of their baby no matter what the stage of pregnancy or the reason for termination.

Stillbirth

In October 1992 the legal definition of a stillbirth was altered from a baby born dead after 28 weeks completed gestation or more to a baby born dead after 24 weeks completed weeks of gestation or more.

In 1992 in England and Wales there were 3160 stillbirths. This included 216 stillbirths of between 24 and 27 completed weeks gestation. The still-birth and perinatal mortality rates were 4.6 and 7.9 per 1000 total births respectively (Office of Population Censuses and Surveys newsletter to the NHS, 1993).

Fifty percent of babies who die *in utero* have no known cause of death. This presents a major obstacle in the grieving process because there is no ready reason or diagnosis. The lack of reason often causes mothers to search or to create a reason and turn the blame inwardly onto themselves or to others.

Giving birth to death is a very complicated and difficult experience but should be remembered as a positive experience. Unfortunately so many complicating factors exist which makes the management of the situation by the interprofessional team extremely difficult. Bourne and Lewis (1984) point out that: 'Careful management helps to preserve the dignity and poignancy of the experience'.

To make the birth a reality is so important for the future mental health of the parents and the key to this is total involvement of the parents and the health care team. Feedback should be given at all stages allowing time for touch, tears, open and honest communication which will help the parents to make the labour and birth a reality. Good communication at this time is imperative and only by listening is it possible to discern the real needs of the parents.

Labour and birth

During labour the woman and her partner must be supported, preferably by the same midwife to aid continuity. The parents must be kept fully informed and their wishes should be fully complied with. The woman should be enabled to be in control and empowered and sustained in order for her to remember that she did give birth. This can be made into a beautiful experience when a caring midwife involves the woman and her partner fully in the event of labour, birth and death.

Many misguided comments are often uttered by members of the hospital team, the relatives and the general public. One woman who was very angry and distressed said:

> If only someone had said that they were sorry; instead I was offered 'You are young, it's your first and you can have another'. But I wanted the baby we had planned and waited two years for.

Creating memories

Women remember their labour and birth and very often the midwife associated with the birth for many years and often more so when a tragedy occurs. It is impossible to take away the pain of a stillbirth; we therefore should work to make the experience as real as is possible by not detracting from what is actually happening. Holding the parents' hands, giving constant feedback about the progress of the labour, providing adequate pain relief in whatever form the woman wishes, helping the woman adopt whatever position she wishes to give birth in, all provide positive memories with which to build a picture of reality to enable grieving to take place. It is so difficult for women to begin grieving during labour and yet death has already occurred.

The professionals involved also need to create good memories for their own esteem to enable them to accept the situation. Guilt, anxiety and remorse are often experienced by the carers.

Following the birth

It is important to encourage the parents to hold the baby, examine the baby, name the baby, take part in washing and dressing the baby. These are all positive actions which contribute to the formation of a basis on which the parents can build and will give positive memories and hopefully encourage grieving. A sensitive and caring midwife can show the parents by example that the baby is real. Sometimes parents may shun the dead baby, possibly owing to the fear of seeing death for the first time. Death is mysterious, even more so when it involves a small and defenceless baby. Anne, whose baby lived for one week, described her experience like this:

> The young doctor asked if we would like to see Philip but we declined the offer – a decision I will regret to my dying day. If only someone could have talked to me, could have explained how important it was to say goodbye to our baby, could have told me how it would help with the grieving process, could have just gently taken me by the hand and supported me.
>
> (SANDS, 1991)

whereas Sue whose baby lived 20 minutes said:

> We were allowed to stay in the delivery room for as long as we wanted, and it was up to us when we wanted to say 'goodbye' to

> Naomi and hand her over to the staff. Peter, Naomi and I were left on our own and the staff just popped their heads round the door occasionally to see if we needed anything. They really got the balance between helpfulness and privacy exactly right.
>
> (SANDS, 1991)

Honesty and openness, listening to the parents' feelings, together with constant information and feedback are required from the midwife and medical staff when caring for a woman whose baby has died before birth or during delivery. It is important to remember that the feelings of isolation, anxiety, hopelessness, guilt, being alone, lacking control and power are shared by all.

Death in the first week of life – early neonatal death

Babies who die in the first week of life are usually ill and have been removed from the mother's care and placed into a neonatal intensive care unit (NICU). There will have been little time since the birth to hold, cuddle and feed the baby. A NICU can be a frightening place, with equipment which make anxiety-provoking noises. The baby may be hidden by tubes and various items of equipment which are helping the baby to stay alive. The parents are afraid to touch the baby, everything becomes unreal and every moment of the day is filled with the thoughts of the baby and its progress: 'Will he/she be all right?', 'Will the baby survive?'.

It is useful to remember the words of Lynn whose baby survived ten hours and 35 minutes:

> When the decision was taken to stop treatment we were given a pleasant quiet room in which to hold and be alone with Kate. Our families were allowed to come and go as they pleased and our minister was able to come and baptize our daughter.
>
> (SANDS, 1991)

Parents may not have seen anyone die before and they may feel frightened. Siblings need to be involved as they can conjure up unreal memories if they are not included in this family situation and may blame themselves for the baby's death.

Complicating factors that may affect all baby deaths

The events of the loss may well be complicated by other factors. When caring for parents who have sustained the loss of a baby it is important to remember that there may well be other obstacles to grieving. The individual may have an inability to cope with emotional distress or conversely be someone who has a very strong and dominant personality who refuses to consider that the grieving process is relevant. There are particular circumstances around the death which may complicate the process, for example, previous unresolved grief, ambivalent feelings towards the dead baby, multiple loss, for example when twins or triplets die or when one twin lives. It is difficult to mourn the death of one baby when parents have to care for and be joyful for the living baby.

In practice there are many examples of this but one in particular comes to mind. Donna and John, whose twin baby died three days after birth following major surgery for a heart defect, had this to say:

> We were so proud to be expecting twins, we planned so much, I was so well, nothing had gone wrong, even the birth was good and then suddenly he was taken away.

Donna suffered for two whole years following the birth and death of Michael. Her general practitioner prescribed antidepressant drugs which repressed her unrelieved feelings even further. He refused her husband's request for Donna to be referred to a counsellor and by the time that she finally managed to find professional help through her own persistent efforts, the whole event had become so complicated, the unravelling so difficult and she felt her personality had been completed shattered. She said:

> My family don't want to listen, they just want the old Donna back. I'm different now, all I want to be is whole again and that means having Michael back to make my family complete.

When she eventually began to come to terms with Michael's death, her thoughts became focused on another pregnancy and she became afraid and needed reassurance and someone to listen to her fears.

Caring for the carers

Staff should be encouraged to share their feelings. Some may have suffered a similar bereavement or have bereavement problems of their own. The stiff upper lip, long associated with caring professionals which encouraged a detached attitude, is no longer acceptable. Sharing in the grief can help the carer as well as the parents and relatives. Recognition of the carers' needs by peers, management and administrative colleagues helps to ease the stress which builds up when caring for women who have experienced a miscarriage, stillbirth or early neonatal death.

There is a need to understand our own feelings and recognize situations which may be particularly difficult for us. Understanding and accepting that there are painful areas is not a weakness but allows us to cope better.

In extreme cases we may even have to recognize that there are times when we cannot cope.

Parkes (1986) and Ovretveit (1986) highlighted the need for support networks during bereavement to ease the process of grief. Communication, mutual support, shared knowledge and skills are absolutely essential. Graham (1991) suggests that lack of communication, power, language and lack of formal training are all complicating factors when bearing bad news. Interprofessional collaboration is essential when devising policies, standards and education and training for health professionals.

A model of good practice

A model of good practice has been formulated by a midwife counsellor (Jones, 1993) which indicates that good communication through a communication network is vital (Fig. 10.2). She states:

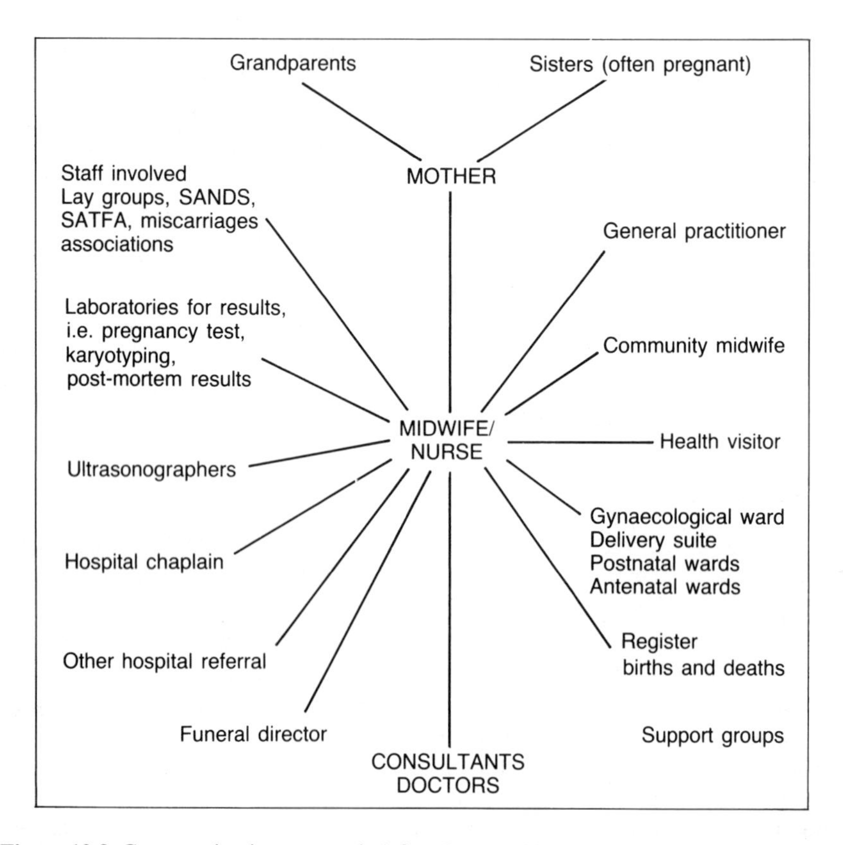

Figure 10.2 Communication network (after Jones, 1993).

> As technology becomes more prominent in care we must provide psychological support according to the needs of women and not as we the professionals assume . . . women and their partners must be allowed to maintain their autonomy by being enabled to make their own decisions.

Principles of good conduct (SANDS, 1991)

SANDS lay down the principles of good conduct which are:

- Parents need information.
- Communication with parents should be clear, sensitive and honest.
- The care given to parents should be responsive to their individual needs and feelings. Parents should be treated with dignity and respect.
- Parents' loss should be recognized and acknowledged, their experiences and feelings validated.
- Parents need to be given time.
- All those involved in the care of bereaved parents should be well informed.
- All those who care for and support bereaved parents should have access to support for themselves.

From many years of experience of working together with women and their partners who have suffered the experience of miscarriage, stillbirth and neonatal death, it has become apparent that listening is the single most important aspect of communication. Women want to talk, to tell and retell their experience, they need this to cleanse themselves of often self-inflicted guilt, doubt, frustration and failure. Most of all they need to share their experience, as do the carers, in order to accept and so be able to say goodbye.

REFERENCES

Alder, S. (1990) Taking children at their word: pain control in paediatrics. *Professional Nurse*, **5**(8), 398–402.

Audit Commission (1993) *A Study of Hospital Services: No. 7, Child, Patients and Hospital Services*, HMSO, London.

Bennett, P. (1984) A care team for terminally ill children. *Nursing Times*, **80**(10), 26–7.

Beyer, J. (1984) *The Oucher: A User's Manual and Technical Report*, The Hospital Play Equipment Co., Evanston.

Bluebond-Langer, M. (1989) Worlds of dying children and their well siblings. *Death Studies*, **13**, 1–16.

Bourne, S. and Lewis, E. (1984) Pregnancy after stillbirth or neonatal death. Psychological risks and management. *Lancet*, **2**(8393), 31–3.

Brady, M. (1993) In *Caring for dying children and their families*, (ed L. Hill), Chapman and Hall, London, p. 127.

Burton, L. (1975) *Family Life of Sick Children*, Routledge and Kegan Paul, Boston.

Cairns, N., Clark, G.M., Smith, S. and Lansky, S. (1979) Adaptation of siblings to childhood cancer. *Journal of Paediatrics*, **95**, 484–7.

Casey, A. (1988) Partnership in practice. *Nursing Times*, **84**(44), 66–8.

Cleary, J., Gray, O., Hall, D., Rowlandson, P., Sainsbury, C. and Davies, M. (1986) Children in hospital. *Archives of Diseases in Childhood*, **61**, 779–87.

Collinge, P. and Stewart, E.D. (1983) Dying children and their families, in *Caring for the Dying Patient and the Family*, 1st edn, (ed. J. Robbins), Harper and Row, London.

Consolvo, C. (1986) Relieving parental anxiety in the care for parent unit. *Journal of Obstetric, Gynaecological and Neonatal Nursing*, **2**, 154–7.

Copsey, M.K. (1981) Time to care. *Nursing Mirror*, **153**(2), 38–40.

Davies, J. (1979) *Death of a Child*, Pitman Medical Publishing Co., London.

Doyle, B. (1987) 'I wish you were dead'. *Nursing Times*, **83**(45), 44–6.

Eland, J. and Anderson, J. (1977) *Pain*, Little, Brown & Co., Boston.

Evans, M. (1977) Caring by parents, in *Child Care – Some Nursing Perspectives*, (ed. A. Glasper), Wolfe Publishing Ltd, London.

Goldman, A., Beardsmore, S. and Hunt, J. (1990) Palliative care for children with cancer – home, hospital or hospice? *Archives of Disease in Childhood*, **65**, 641–3.

Gonda, T. and Ruark, J. (1984) *Dying Dignified. The Health Professional Guide to Care*, Addison Wesley, Menlo Park CA.

Graham, S.B. (1991) Structured analysis of the physician–midwife interaction in an obstetric programme (research study in USA). *Social Science and Medicine*, **32**(8), 931–42.

Harris, P. (1981) How parents feel. *Nursing Times*, **77**(42), 1803–4.

Hill, L. (1993) *Caring for Dying Children and their Families*, Chapman & Hall, London.

Hunt, J. (1990) Symptom care of the child with cancer. *Nursing Times*, **86**(10), 72–3.

Jennings, P. (1992) Coping strategies for mothers. *Paediatric Nursing*, **4**(9), 24–6.

Jolly, J. (1981) *The Other Side of Paediatrics: A Guide to the Everyday Care of Sick Children*, Macmillan, London.

Jolly, J. (1989) *Missed Beginnings. Death Before Life has been Established*, The Lisa Sainsbury Foundation, Austen Cornish, London.

Jones, P. (1993) *A Model of Good Practice*, Luton & Dunstable NHS Trust (unpublished).

Judd, D. (1993) Communicating with dying children, in *Death, Dying and Bereavement*, (eds D. Dickenson and M. Johnson), Sage Publications Ltd, London.

Kohner, N. and Henley, A. (1991) *When A Baby Dies*, Pandora, London.

Lansdown, R. (1980) *More than Sympathy*, Tavistock, London.

Lansdown, R. and Benjamin, G. (1988) The development of the concept of death in children aged 5–9 years. *Childcare and Development*, **11**, 13–20.

Lauer, M., Mulhern, R., Wallskog, J. and Camitta, B. (1983) A comparison study of parental adaptation following a child's death at home or in hospital. *Paediatrics*, **71**(1), 107–12.

MacDonald, A. (1988) A model for children's nursing. *Nursing Times*, **84**, 52–5.

McAll, K. (1982) *Healing the Family Tree*, Sheldon, London.

Muller, D., Harris, P., Wattle, L. and Taylor, J. (1992) *Nursing Children – Psychology, Research & Practice*, 2nd edn, Chapman & Hall, London.

Ovretveit, J. (1986) *Organization Of Multidisciplinary Community Teams*, Brunel University, Middlesex.

Parkes, C.M. (1986) *Bereavement; Studies of Grief in Adult Life*, Penguin, Harmondsworth.

Piaget, J. (1954) *The Construction of Reality in the Child*, 2nd edn, Basic Books, New York.

Platt, H. (1959) *The Welfare of Children in Hospital.* Report of the Committee on Child Health Services, HMSO, London.

Reilly, T., Hasazi, J. and Bond, L. (1983) Children's conceptions of death and personal mortality. *Journal of Paediatric Psychology*, **8**, 21–31.

Rodin, J. (1983) *Will This Hurt?* RCN, London.

Sadler, S. (1988) Being there. *Nursing Times*, **84**(34), 19.

Saunders, B. (1982) Staff support. *Nursing*, **1**(34), 1498–9.

Siedel, M. (1981) Death education – a continuing process for nurses. *Topics in Clinical Nursing*, **3**(3), 87–9.

Spence, J. (1947) The care of children in hospital. *British Medical Journal*, **1**, 125–30.

Stillbirth and Neonatal Death Society (1991) *Miscarriage, Stillbirth and Neonatal Death: Guidelines for Professionals*, SANDS, London.

Swaffield, L. (1988) Sharing the load. *Nursing Times*, **84**(36), 24–26.

Vidovich, M. (1980) Caring for kids – death in the ICU. *Australian Nurses Journal*, **9**, 43–4.

Webb, N., Hull, D. and Madeley, R. (1985) Care by parents in hospital. *British Medical Journal*, **291**, 176–7.

Whitting, M. (1990) Home truths. *Nursing Times*, **85**(14), 74–5.

Wright, B. (1991) *Sudden Death*, Churchill Livingstone, Edinburgh.

11 Care of the dying patient with AIDS

INTRODUCTION

HIV infection has been described as the greatest new public health challenge this century (DoH, 1993). The numbers of people infected with HIV are steadily rising and with this the demands placed on local statutory and voluntary services who provide care will increase.

People are infected with HIV in every country in the world. It affects a diversity of people, men, women and children. The concept of high risk groups is outdated despite efforts by the media to perpetuate this. The focus for HIV prevention initiatives is largely based on high-risk activities rather than particular high-risk groups.

Sadly, issues of fear, ignorance, prejudice and discrimination surround the subject of HIV and AIDS. As a result of this many people with HIV do not divulge their HIV status openly for fear of recrimination and victimization. Many have concerns about confidentiality and the responses of others when they learn of their HIV status. It is vital that the professionals involved in their care ensure that the patient's right to confidentiality is upheld as far as possible.

Many individuals with HIV must learn to cope with the uncertainty which continually overshadows their HIV infection. The path of the disease is never predictable as it affects individuals in many different ways and for those who live with HIV, it poses many questions which professionals cannot answer. How long will they remain healthy? Which of the many HIV related illnesses will they develop? When will they receive their first AIDS diagnosis?

The nursing care of a patient with end-stage HIV disease should be that which is offered to any dying patient. Health care professionals must respond positively to the challenge of HIV/AIDS by developing accurate knowledge of the disease and attaining the skills necessary to provide high quality care for people affected by it.

WHAT IS HIV?

Transmission

HIV stands for human immunodeficiency virus. It is transmitted in the following ways:

- sexually, via contact with infected blood, semen, cervical and vaginal fluids;
- following transfusion of blood or blood products from a donor infected with HIV;
- injecting substance misuse and contamination with infected blood through sharing needles and syringes;
- following organ transplants or artificial insemination by donor semen;
- transplacental and perinatal transmission.

There are no documented cases of HIV transmission through social contact. Historically a source of concern for health care workers caring for someone with HIV infection was the likelihood of transmission occurring during clinical procedures. Although there have been some incidents of health care workers becoming HIV positive as a result of occupational exposure (most of these being needlestick injuries) the rate of transmission via this route is estimated to be only 0.3% in comparison with the estimated 30% chance following exposure to hepatitis B.

HOW HIV AFFECTS THE BODY

Once inside the body the virus searches for cells for which it has an affinity. These include certain cells in the central nervous system and commonly the T4 lymphocytes or helper cells which play a vital role in the body's immune system and its defence against infection. Once the virus enters the cell it may lie dormant for a number of years (on average 10–12). During this time the person may remain relatively healthy but is able to transmit the virus to others. The virus remains dormant within the cell until it is activated, possibly by an infection or some other yet unknown stimulant. This triggers the virus to replicate and these new virus cells bud out of the host cell and go on to infect other cells. Eventually the T4 cell dies.

A blood test which measures the amount of T4 cells in the body and thus gives an indication of how the immune system is functioning is known as a T4 (or CD4) count. This is a useful marker for physicians and can be used as a guide to introducing specific primary prophylaxis, i.e. a patient with a T4 count of 200 or less is at risk of developing *pneumocystis carinii* pneumonia and should be offered prophylactic therapy.

INFECTION CONTROL

The use of universal precautions as standard practice serves as a valuable and necessary infection control measure. It is unreliable and hazardous to adopt special infection control procedures only for those patients who are known to be HIV or hepatitis B positive. The British Medical Association (1993) endorses this with the statement:

> While special precautions are recommended when treating patients known to be carrying bloodborne viruses such as hepatitis B and HIV, many patients will not have been identified, and the only safe approach is to assume that any patient may be a carrier.

The following are basic principles of infection control and should be adopted when caring for any patient, regardless of their HIV status.

1. A disposable plastic apron and good quality plastic or latex gloves should be worn when there is likely to be contact with a patient's blood and body fluids. These should be discarded following contact with each patient.
2. Masks and eye protection should only be used when carrying out or assisting with invasive procedures during which splashing of body fluids may occur. They may also be used if the patient is coughing excessively.
3. Cover any cuts or abrasions on the hands with a waterproof dressing.
4. If gloved hands are contaminated with blood or body fluids, they should be washed immediately and thoroughly with soap and warm water or Hibiscrub if this is available.
5. Needles and syringes should be disposable. After use the needle and syringe should be disposed of in a sharps bin as a completed unit. Never resheath the needle.
6. Spillage of blood or body fluids should be covered with disinfectant granules, such as Presept, left for a few minutes and then carefully wiped up with disposable paper towels. Spillage in the home should be cleaned with a 1 in 10 solution of fresh strong bleach. For spillage onto carpets or upholstery, mop up excess fluid and sponge area with warm water and detergent.
7. Members of staff who are immunodeficient/compromised either through illness or therapy or suffering from exfoliative skin conditions should seek the advice of the Occupational Health Department before nursing patients with HIV (Sims and Moss, 1991).

AN AIDS DIAGNOSIS

AIDS stands for Acquired Immune Deficiency Syndrome. As a person's immune system becomes impaired by HIV, they become more susceptible to developing a range of illnesses or infections. These may be considered relatively uncommon in the general population or may be seen as minor problems in people with an intact immune system. An AIDS diagnosis is specified as the development of an opportunistic infection, a malignancy associated with immunosuppression or neurological impairment as a direct result of the infiltration of HIV on the central nervous system. Other AIDS defining diagnoses include profound weight loss resulting in extensive muscle wasting.

Clinical staging for HIV infection (Europe)

Clinical stage 1

- Asymptomatic
- Persistent generalized lymphadenopathy

Clinical stage 2

- Weight loss <10% of body weight
- Minor skin/mucous membrane infections
- Herpes zoster (in the last five years)
- Recurrent upper respiratory tract infections

Clinical stage 3

- Weight loss >10% of body weight
- Unexplained pyrexia, intermittent/constant for longer than one month
- Oral candidia
- Oral hairy leucoplakia
- Pulmonary tuberculosis within the past year
- Severe bacterial infections

Clinical stage 4 (AIDS)

- HIV wasting syndrome
- *Pneumocystis carinii* pneumonia
- Toxoplasmosis
- Cryptosporidiosis with diarrhoea for longer than one month
- Cryptococcosis, extrapulmonary
- Cytomegalovirus other than liver, spleen and lymph nodes

- Herpes simplex virus for longer than one month
- Progressive multifocal leukoencephalopathy
- Candida affecting the oesophagus, trachea, bronchi or lungs
- A typical mycobacteriosis, disseminated. MAI
- Non-typhoid salmonella septicaemia
- Extrapulmonary tuberculosis
- Lymphoma
- Kaposi's sarcoma
- HIV encephalopathy (AIDS related dementia)
- Pulmonary TB
- CIN
- Pulmonary bacterial infections

COMMON OPPOTUNISTIC INFECTIONS

Pneumocystis carinii pneumonia (PCP)

PCP was originally thought to be caused by a protozoan but is now thought to be caused by fungi. It is present as a normal flora in most adults which rarely causes disease unless an individual becomes immunosuppressed. It is the most common opportunistic infection seen in patients with HIV and approximately 80% of patients will develop this in the course of their illness (Barter, Barton and Gazzard, 1993).

Symptoms

The onset of PCP is usually insidious with patients complaining of shortness of breath over a period of 3–4 weeks. Other symptoms may include chest pain, fever/rigours and cyanosis. Alternatively some patients may present with a much shorter history and show signs of acute respiratory distress.

Diagnosis

A diagnosis of PCP is made after a series of clinical investigations. These include:

- chest X-ray;
- arterial blood gases;
- lung function tests;
- sputum specimens;
- bronchoscopy.

Treatment

This is often initiated prior to confirmation of sputum specimen results. Treatment options include either inhaled, oral or intravenous antibiotic therapy depending on the severity of the patient's symptoms.

Choice of treatment options available for PCP:

- oral or intravenous cotrimoxazole;
- inhaled or intravenous pentamidine;
- oral or intravenous clindamycin with primaquine;
- oral dapsone with or without trimethoprim.

In addition patients may require supportive oxygen therapy and, in severe cases of respiratory distress, may need intravenous corticosteroids.

John, 31, has been HIV positive for six years and was admitted to the ward with a three week history of breathlessness on exertion, fevers and a dry, unproductive cough. This was John's first admission to hospital for an HIV related illness and his partner remained with him on the ward. A diagnosis of PCP was made following a bronchoscopy. John's needs were assessed by his named nurse and after discussion with him a plan of care was devised.

Case Study

1. John was encouraged to adopt an upright sitting position, well supported by pillows. It was explained that this would assist in improving respiratory function.
2. John was given continuous oxygen therapy to relieve hypoxaemia via a Ventimask or nasal cannulae. This caused him to have a dry mouth, so frequent mouth care was performed by the nursing staff and his partner. Ice cubes and regular cool drinks were offered to quench his thirst and maintain adequate fluid intake.
3. John was understandably anxious about his first time in hospital and his first AIDS diagnosis. The nurses caring for him offered support and reassurance to both John and his partner. He was given time to discuss and explore his feelings about various issues such as what an AIDS diagnosis means, planning for the future and measures to maximize his health.
4. John and his partner were actively encouraged to participate in decisions made about his care. Clear explanations were given for nursing and medical interventions which helped reduce their anxiety and allowed John to maintain control over his illness.
5. John was commenced on intravenous cotrimoxazole as treatment for his PCP. As a result he experienced side effects of nausea and

vomiting. To combat this he was given an antiemetic prior to administration of his treatment. This was successful and John completed a course of treatment which lasted three weeks.

6. Before John's discharge it was explained to him that the PCP could return and so it was necessary for him to continue with medication as prophylaxis to avoid this.

OTHER COMMON OPPORTUNISTIC INFECTIONS

Cryptosporidiosis

Cryptosporidium is a parasite which largely affects the small intestine. It is a common pathogen in the general population and in immunocompromised individuals can cause serious illness.

Symptoms

These include abdominal cramps, nausea and vomiting, fevers and diarrhoea resulting in weight loss. The severity of the symptoms can vary between patients depending on their immune function. For some, it may cause occasional bouts of diarrhoea, for others it can cause large volumes of watery diarrhoea several times a day.

Diagnosis

This is made by examination of stool cultures or biopsies of the gastrointestinal mucosa.

Treatment

This is generally for symptomatic purposes. There is ongoing research into various treatment options but as yet there have been few conclusive results available. Drugs given to control the diarrhoea include Imodium, Lomotil, codeine phosphate and morphine.

Nutritional support is extremely important in an effort to stabilize the patient's weight. Dietetic advice should be sought early on. Nutritional supplements as well as regular snacks between meals should be offered. Enteral feeding may be considered.

Cryptosporidiosis causes some of the most undignified symptoms which can have a direct effect on the patient's psychological state. Their embarrassment and loss of self-esteem, together with the limitations these symptoms place on their quality of life, should be sensitively addressed. The nursing care should aim to preserve the patient's dignity and self-esteem as far as possible, incorporating practical measures to alleviate distressing symptoms.

Cytomegalovirus (CMV)

Cytomegalovirus can affect the gastrointestinal tract causing colitis and ulceration, the lungs causing pneumonitis and, most commonly, the eyes leading to retinitis.

CMV Retinitis

This usually occurs in patients who have already had other AIDS related illnesses or who are severely immunosuppressed. The eyes are often examined at each follow-up appointment as untreated CMV retinitis may result in blindness.

Symptoms

Patients often present with a history of gradual visual blurring, seeing 'floaters' or partial or complete loss of visual fields.

Diagnosis

Diagnosis is made after ophthalmic examination where white areas and haemorrhages can be seen on the retina.

Treatment

Once a diagnosis is made, treatment is initiated promptly. This is in the form of intravenous ganciclovir or Foscarnet for a period of 14–21 days. Treatment aims to deactivate the CMV and generally will not improve already impaired vision. Once patients have completed this course of treatment, it is essential to continue with a maintenance therapy regime in an intravenous form for the rest of their lives. Recurrence of CMV retinitis can be common despite prophylaxis.

Long term therapy

Patients are offered the choice of having either a Hickman line or Portacath inserted to provide long term venous access. The patient and/or carer are taught how to administer the medication and how to care for the intravenous line. After discharge the district nurse can offer support and supervision or can take on this role if the patient is unable to do so.

The presence of a permanent intravenous line can serve as a constant reminder to the patient of their HIV infection and can affect their perception of their body image. Combined with the daily routine of injecting the medication, which can be time consuming, comes the restrictions this may impose on their daily activities. Measures to simplify the administration of intravenous drugs at home include portable prefilled infusion devices which are inconspicuous and easy to use. These devices also assist in reducing the risk of introducing infection into the line. The potential risk of systemic infection is increased in HIV positive patients who are already immunosuppressed.

HIV RELATED MALIGNANCIES

The development of malignancies is a complication of a failing immune system. The most common malignancies seen in HIV disease are Kaposi's sarcoma and non-Hodgkin's lymphoma.

Kaposi's sarcoma (KS)

Before the advent of HIV disease, KS was largely seen to affect middle-aged to elderly men of Jewish, East European or Mediterranean descent. In patients with HIV, it is most commonly seen in homosexual or bisexual men. There remains some speculation as to the reason for this.

Symptoms

Patients may discover small raised purplish skin lesions which are initially painless. They can present on any part of the body and in later stages of the illness may disseminate to involve the lungs, the gastrointestinal tract and the lymphatic system.

Diagnosis

Diagnosis is made by performing a biopsy of the lesion.

Treatment

Treatment does not improve overall survival or the rate of appearance of new lesions. It is useful for cosmetic purposes and for the relief of local troublesome oedematous or painful lesions. The options are discussed with the patient and fall into two categories – local radiotherapy or systemic chemotherapy. A problem associated with administering cytotoxic therapy to HIV positive patients is that this can lead to further immunosuppression and as a result, the risk of developing other opportunistic infections.

Cutaneous KS lesions can commonly affect the face and other areas visible to others. Camouflage make-up can be used to cover the lesions. Patients who have facial lesions may be conscious that this is a blatant sign to others of their HIV infection and consequently this may compound their feelings of loss of body image.

Non-Hodgkin's lymphoma

In HIV disease, these are usually high grade B cell lymphomas. Most frequently affected sites include the central nervous system, bone marrow, GI tract, liver and lymph nodes.

Symptoms

These vary as to the site of the lymphoma. They may include fever, weight loss, diarrhoea, GI bleeding, an enlarging mass and neurological symptoms.

Diagnosis

Again this will depend on the suspected site for the lymphoma. A range of clinical investigations may be performed including examinations of biopsies of the affected organ.

Treatment

This may be in the form of combination chemotherapy and radiotherapy.

HIV encephalopathy (AIDS related dementia)

HIV encephalopathy occurs as a direct result of the virus replicating in the brain tissue. It leads to a progressive loss of cognitive and behavioural function.

Approximately 6–10% of people with AIDS will go on to develop dementia. Its onset is insidious and it commonly manifests in the final stages of the disease.

Symptoms

Early signs may include short term memory loss, loss of concentration, periods of confusion, personality and behavioural changes. As this progresses it leads to more increased neurological impairment characterized by tremor, ataxia, limb weakness, loss of coordination eventually leading to paralysis, incontinence and death.

Diagnosis

A CT or MRI scan is performed which may reveal severe widespread cerebral atrophy with destruction of the white matter in the brain.

Treatment

The use of AZT has produced a significant improvement in patients with AIDS dementia by improving neurological function in the short term and slowing down further deterioration.

The prospect of developing AIDS dementia is one which many people with HIV fear the most out of all HIV related conditions. The possibility of losing one's faculties and having to become fully dependent on those around one is distressing to imagine and difficult for all involved to deal with. Occasionally, as with any dementia, patients affected may become verbally and physically aggressive, lashing out at their loved ones and others around them. It is vital that there are strong support networks established for the partners and loved ones caring for a patient. When the care is based in the community, the partner and loved ones should be offered support and assistance in the care from both professional and voluntary agencies. The opportunity for the carer to have a respite break from this caring role should also be offered regularly, whether this is in the form of some time for the patient in a residential setting or time out for the carer knowing that their loved one is being cared for by others at home.

POINTS TO CONSIDER WHEN CARING FOR PEOPLE WITH HIV/AIDS

HIV infection can result in a multisystems disease. Often patients who are in the end stage of their illness have had several opportunistic infections or HIV related illnesses. As a result of this they may be on a range of different drugs for a variety of reasons, i.e. prophylaxis therapy, antiretrovirals (AZT, DDI) and drugs to control symptoms. Due to the complexity of the disease it is common for patients to have a variety of distressing symptoms which need controlling. These might include such things as weight loss, night sweats, anorexia, diarrhoea, neuropathic pain, nausea and vomiting (which may be induced by multiple drug therapy).

Where to care?

Many people with HIV have chosen to base their inpatient and outpatient care at large specialist treatment centres. The reasons for this include the anonymity this brings and the level of specialist care and knowledge at these perceived centres of excellence. As acute and community HIV/AIDS services continue to develop on a local level, more patients are electing to be treated closer to their home. This benefits the patients and carers not only in terms of convenience but it also allows them to establish trusting relationships with local health care professionals. This involvement from an early stage allows the relationship to develop before the patient enters the terminal stage and wishes to die at home. The use of generic services to provide care rather than specialist services can assist in normalizing and demystifying the concept of HIV/AIDS. Ultimately, the choice of where to base their care should rest with the patient and this should be respected.

A model of care

A multidisciplinary, multiagency approach to caring for people with HIV infection serves as an appropriate model which aims to address the many and varied needs of the individual. The skill and expertise made available to the patient in this approach can ensure that their holistic needs are met. The patient's expressed wishes should remain the focus of the care at all times. A coordinated core package with good communication between all involved can assist in monitoring the level of input by each agency and avoid duplication of services which might serve to confuse the patient and carers.

Active versus palliative

The decision on when to stop active treatment is always a difficult one to make and in the case of people with AIDS, is never clear cut. Discussions around this should ideally occur when the patient is able to participate in the decision making process. When a person is nearing the end stage of their illness, it is vital that the health care professionals are honest and open, outlining their probable prognosis if this is appropriate, the pros and cons of further treatment and the effect this may have on their quality of life in the future. This can ensure that decisions are made from an informed position. Patients may elect to continue with prophylaxis therapy but decide not to have active treatment if any new infection occurs, i.e. they may continue with intravenous ganciclovir for CMV retinitis to prevent the onset of blindness but not be treated for a new bout of PCP.

Living will

This is a document which ensures that the patient's wishes concerning treatment are known when the time comes that they are unable to make decisions for themselves, for example when they become unconscious or develop AIDS related dementia. The living will was devised by the Terence Higgins Trust in conjunction with King's College, London. It is drawn up by the patient in discussion with their doctor and can be kept in their medical notes as a reference. Although this document is not legally binding, it can be a useful guide for physicians to identify the patient's wishes if these circumstances arise.

Hospice care

Until recently, the palliative care options available to people with HIV were fairly limited. They could be cared for at home which continues to become more popular with patients. Some choose to return to their acute treatment centre to die, others may wish to be admitted to one of the specialist HIV/AIDS hospices. Many generic hospices have re-examined their admission criteria and now offer respite, convalescent and terminal care to people with AIDS.

Complementary therapies

As the conventional medical approach to HIV and AIDS cannot yet offer all the answers, patients may wish to explore alternative avenues. Many HIV positive patients choose to use complementary therapies often in conjunction with their conventional treatment. An obvious advantage in most complementary therapies is the important part they play in stress reduction, as well as the other benefits they might have, such as enhancing the immune system and improving the patient's quality of life. As there have been few trials to evaluate the effectiveness of complementary therapies this has led to scepticism among some medical staff about their use. However many physicians caring for people with AIDS recognize their value and importance to the patients and encourage the use of these therapies in the acute hospital setting.

Support for staff

The advent of HIV/AIDS has challenged the conventional doctor/nurse–patient relationship. Often people with HIV are well informed about their illness, sometimes more so than the professionals caring for them and many request full involvement in their care. This often results in a more open, honest and trusting relationship between professional and patient with both working in partnership. Multiple bereavements as a result of caring for people with AIDS can have a profound effect on the professionals working in this field and should be addressed. Nurses may find themselves caring for people faced with a terminal illness who are of a similar age to themselves; they are caring for their peer group.

Nursing people with AIDS can prove stressful and so the need for staff support must be acknowledged. Staff may find different methods of support beneficial, whether this is offered informally by peers of colleagues or formally in the form of supervision or support groups facilitated by an appropriately experienced counsellor.

Very often nursing staff have known a patient for a number of months or even years, possibly as a result of the patient's numerous admissions to hospital. When a patient dies the nursing staff should be allowed to attend the funeral if they wish. This acts as a method of completing their care.

CARE STUDY

The following care study has been included to bring together the various principles of care described in this chapter.

Tom

Tom is a 31 year old man who was diagnosed HIV positive in March 1986. He met Lisa in July 1987 and they married shortly after. Since their relationship began they always practised safe sex.

Tom attended his local genitourinary medicine clinic for follow-up appointments on a 3-monthly basis where he was offered support and advice from the multidisciplinary team there. Despite minor illnesses and infections, Tom continued to enjoy his work as a teacher in a primary school. His work colleagues were unaware of his status.

In January 1991 Tom was admitted to an acute medical ward with PCP. This was successfully treated and he returned to work after a convalescent break.

As time wore on Tom became conscious of his changing body image, his weight was steadily falling and his energy levels were low. He felt tired most of the time and he was concerned that his colleagues may begin to question his illness or even suspect his HIV status. After discussion with Lisa, he decided to contact a social worker to find out his benefit entitlement prior to resigning from his job on medical grounds.

Now in receipt of full benefits he maintained contact with the social worker who continued to provide support to both him and Lisa. The local clinical nurse specialist (CNS) for HIV/AIDS assisted in coordinating Tom's care at home and she saw him regularly to assess his symptoms and to provide emotional support. Shortly after Tom had given up work he and Lisa decided to spend some of their savings on the holiday that they had always promised themselves. On their return they both felt that this would be a good time to make arrangements for the future, so both decided to make a will.

In March 1992, following a 3-week history of intermittent abdominal pain and diarrhoea, Tom was diagnosed as having cryptosporidiosis. His GP prescribed codeine phosphate to control the diarrhoea and help alleviate the stomach cramps. The CNS introduced a district nurse to Tom, who subsequently visited him regularly. After discussion with Tom, she arranged for a commode and Inco pads to be delivered for days when his diarrhoea was particularly bad. Measures on handling soiled linen and waste were discussed with Tom and Lisa. It was explained that any soiled linen could be laundered in a washing machine on a hot cycle. Soiled dressings and waste would need to be placed in a yellow clinical waste bag and collected by the refuse disposal services. Gloves were provided for dealing with blood and body fluids.

The CNS continued to provide advice, support and guidance for the district nurse who cared for Tom.

Some months later, Tom complained of blurred vision in his right eye. His GP promptly referred him to an ophthalmologist who diagnosed CMV retinitis. A Hickman line was inserted in hospital and intravenous ganciclovir commenced. Lisa and Tom were taught how to care for the Hickman line by the ward staff and they supervised Tom in administering his i.v. drugs until he was confident and competent to do this independently. When he was discharged, the district nurse visited Tom daily, initially to observe his injection technique and offer support. As Tom's sight and coordination deteriorated the district nurse offered to take on this role which Tom and Lisa agreed to.

As Tom's general condition deteriorated further he began to talk openly about his fears around death and dying. He was not afraid of death itself but rather the mode of dying. He was assured by the GP and district nurse that everything would be done to make him as comfortable as possible. Tom had made the decision to have no further active treatment, but to continue with his i.v. ganciclovir as he feared going blind in his final days due to CMV retinitis. All his other medication was geared to symptom control. He expressed a wish to remain at home until he died. He discussed his funeral arrangements with Lisa and requested which type of music he wanted played and the type of service. He also discussed this with his local parish priest who was to conduct the service.

Tom's parents and his two sisters lived nearby and had been aware of his HIV status since his first hospital admission for PCP. They continued to be very supportive and assisted Lisa in caring for Tom. At this difficult time, informal support was offered by all those directly involved in Tom's care. Lisa attended a carers support group run by the local HIV/AIDS voluntary agency. She found it very beneficial to be able to talk openly with others in a similar situation as herself. The volunteer group also offered a sitting service for times when Lisa needed some respite from her caring role and when Tom's family were unable to stay with him. A home help was arranged who visited several times a week and carried out practical tasks in the home, so that Lisa and Tom's family could spend more time with him.

On 10th June 1993, Tom became unconscious and needed full nursing care. The district nurse visited three times a day to ensure that Tom remained comfortable and pain free and offered support to Lisa and the family who continued to perform the majority of his care. Tom's pain relief was adjusted as necessary and administered via a syringe driver. In the early hours of 15th June, Tom died peacefully with Lisa and his family at his side.

After death

The district nurse arrived early that morning and contacted the GP who came to certify the death. The GP then contacted the undertaker and asked them to provide a plastic body bag. The cause of death on the death certificate was stated as bronchopneumonia. The GP was aware that stating the cause of death as AIDS might cause undue distress to the relatives as the certificate is a public document and anyone can have access to this. By marking the certificate appropriately, thus inviting the coroner to request further information if required, this assisted in preserving confidentiality.

Lisa and Tom's family were allowed to spend time alone with him to say their goodbyes. The district nurse and Lisa then performed the Last Offices. Tom was dressed in his favourite tracksuit and then placed in a body bag. Some of Tom's family and friends wished to see him whilst he lay in the chapel of rest before the funeral. The body bag was unzipped to expose Tom's face and the body bag was covered discreetly with a sheet.

The funeral

Some of the health care professionals that had been involved in Tom's care attended his funeral which was conducted just as he had wished.

Bereavement care

The CNS and social worker continued to see Lisa and members of Tom's family on several occasions after his death. Lisa continued to have involvement with the local volunteer group and after some time decided to become a volunteer for the group herself so as to offer support to others affected by HIV/AIDS.

REFERENCES

Barter, G., Barton, S. and Gazzard, B. (1993) *HIV and AIDS – Your Questions Answered*, Churchill Livingstone, Edinburgh.

British Medical Association (1993) *A Code of Practice for the Safe Use and Disposal of Sharps*, BMA, London.

Department of Health (1993) *The Health of the Nation – Key Area Handbook 'HIV/AIDS and Sexual Health'*, HMSO, London.

Sims, R. and Moss, V. (1991) *Terminal Care for People with AIDS*, Edward Arnold, London.

12 Meeting the needs of staff

Caring for the dying person and offering support to bereaved relatives is demanding and stressful, as claimed by Farrell (1992). He goes on to say that 'It can also be a growing and rewarding experience, provided the required supportive mechanisms are available and utilized by the professional carer'. While the greatest input in the terminal phase of a person's illness will come from the nursing staff, as stated by Braun and Katz (1989), all the caring professions will at times be involved.

JUNIOR STAFF AND STUDENTS

As with many other spheres of work, care for the dying carries its own type of emotional stress. Often the more junior staff and students have the closest relationships with patients. This can have advantages in terms of job satisfaction (Eakes, 1990), but it can also be a potential cause of strain. When allocating students of whatever discipline, this latter point should be borne in mind. Adequate support and supervision by senior staff should be readily available at all times, not only because the patient's condition may change quickly and unexpectedly but also to support the student emotionally.

STRESS

Tolerance to stress is an individual matter; a particular situation may be very stressful to one person but apparently have little or no effect on others. Continuing stress is a sign that the situation being endured is excessive and can be a danger signal that actual illness will occur. Stress is not of itself a disease but a protective response which can be used, such as grief, as noted by Fisher (1991). Anger and fear can also be used when there are threats to physical and psychological well-being. It is the prolongation of these responses that is the danger, resulting in intolerable strain.

FEELINGS

To be effective, staff need to be aware of their own feelings and to have a knowledge of their inner strengths and weaknesses. McKerrow (1991) believes that there is a connection between the psychological care of patients and the feelings of the caregivers. After an upsetting experience, staff should find someone to talk to but should in turn be willing to listen, otherwise someone else's stress level may be increased. This type of informed support can take place at work or later with family or friends. For some people, if they are feeling tense, such actions as stretching, yawning or loosening the shoulder and neck muscles by gentle movements will aid relaxation.

Crying

The use of emotional discharges such as crying, laughing or 'storming' are means towards a natural healing process. Neuberger (1986), in her article 'A Crying Shame', says that 'Most dying patients want their nurses to share their anger and then their grief'. She goes on to say that there is 'nothing unprofessional about it – the professionalism lies in being able to weep, and then to take control again and offer practical assistance'.

BEREAVEMENT

Staff need to recognize their own bereavement and sense of loss and hopefully to seek help. Eakes (1990) finds it necessary to say goodbye both to the person who has died and to the family. She would not find it as useful to attend the funeral. Others claim that being present at a funeral, when it is appropriate, provides a proper conclusion to the relationship. It is worth acknowledging that these bereavement visits can be therapeutic to the staff member as well as to the relative and this is quite acceptable.

GRIEF

Fisher (1991) poses the question of whether or not staff grief in palliative care can be turned into healing and growth. A major emotional investment may have been made in the dying person in the form of psychosocial, spiritual, symptom control or physical care. Then dressing a fungating wound may have been carried out with diligence. As with any investment, it may yield dividends, but at a cost.

When a person dies there can be unanswered questions such as 'Could I have done more?', 'Could the patient have been more comfortable or more at peace?'. It is when these issues are explored in conjunction with others that self-growth can take place.

OWN MORTALITY

Sooner or later the question of one's own mortality will come before the conscientious health care worker. It may be raised as an issue at a staff seminar or may come from within, through the daily contact with death and dying. RCN Cancer Nursing Society members (Scott, 1993) heard that faith makes carers better communicators.

SUPPORT GROUPS

Support groups are tried by many units and take several different forms. It may be compulsory for staff to attend or they may be held away from the workplace and staff are invited to join. A good starting point is when there is a felt need and a group is initiated by the staff themselves. A facilitator may be engaged or a leader may be chosen from within. To be successful, staff members need to make a commitment to each other and to the group, as described by Penson (1990). Ironically such group work can cause stress and therefore needs constant evaluation.

COMPLAINTS

It is widely recognized that even with the best of intentions, things may go wrong. One is reminded that health care workers are human too and not always perfect. Michael Quoist (1968) offers some consolation when he says 'Be yourself, others need you just as the Lord has willed you to be'.

Hospice workers and hopefully most people in the caring professions receive an abundance of praise and gratitude for the services they render. To graciously accept such comments a person needs to be spiritually and emotionally mature. However, we are moving into a legalistic age and with a better informed general public plus the reaction to a bereavement, complaints are more likely to be voiced if not also written. For the dedicated worker this can cause much distress, as noted by Farrell (1992).

Management need to be wise and prudent in how they approach their staff concerning a complaint, which may reveal that a staff member is suffering from 'burnout', as discovered by Braun and Katz (1989). In such a case there is need for immediate support which may take the form of personal counselling. Sometimes a change of job is the answer but, regrettably, talented and sensitive people can be lost forever to their chosen profession because of insufficient awareness and help from others at a crucial time. No-one is exempt from this potential hazard and each person should be aware of their own vulnerability and that of their colleagues.

STAFF MORALE

When a unit is found to be under pressure it is important for management to address the question of staff morale as recommended by Owen (1991). Staff need to feel cared for and not simply by increasing the staff establishment, although in some instances this may be part of the answer. Lowered morale or burnout can cause staff to become detached and distance themselves from patients and colleagues, which can produce a chain of negative reactions.

GOALS

The present climate of standard setting can be used to the advantage of staff morale. When realistic goals are set and achieved these can increase job satisfaction. Eakes (1990) explains that a goal can be reached even though a death was involved.

WORKING ENVIRONMENT

Unless the place of work is a hospice or other purpose-built unit, the environmental conditions may be far from ideal for the care of a dying patient. This in itself will be a strain for staff even though the patient and their family will feel more than compensated for any inconvenience of surroundings by a high quality of personal care. A major problem may be lack of a room set aside for use when privacy is essential. Medical and nursing staff frequently need to talk with close relatives or a patient; families want to talk together and relax when spending long periods with a dying relative.

Health care workers also need some privacy during or after an emotionally traumatic time. Ingenuity can usually produce a temporary haven and a short break away from the ward for a cup of coffee will be appreciated and enables the person to recover their equilibrium before resuming care of the patients.

Staff caring for patients in their own homes learn to accept that even though the physical environment might be considered less than ideal, being at home will far outweigh any inconvenience. This will also be the viewpoint of the family where home care is also their wish, as long as they have adequate professional support.

PERSONAL RESPONSIBILITY

All staff who are in continuous or frequent involvement with dying patients should be particularly aware of the need to balance their professional life with family, friends and recreation. Managers will be mindful of the need to see that they and their staff have reasonable off-duty arrangements and the occasional long break.

PROFESSIONAL PREPARATION AND CONTINUING EDUCATION

It is interesting to note that Stoller (1988) found trained registered nurses' unease in interaction with the dying patient and their family increases with experience rather than decreases. If this is so for this group of health professionals then it is probably true for others and therefore how important it is for those who come to work in a hospice setting and into the Macmillan service that there is a period of orientation. Therefore a well-planned programme of induction is essential to enable staff to adjust to their role and feel that they can effectively give care.

Registered nurses are encouraged to participate in the ENB 931 Continuing Care of the Dying Patient and the Family course which enables them to extend their expertise wherever they are working with the dying person.

For others who wish to expand their knowledge and practice, opportunities are now available to undertake multidisciplinary courses at diploma or degree level. The shared learning experience, plus the time to explore the views of others arising from such programmes, are of considerable value.

Harris (1988) found that when education and support needs are addressed, those working with the dying patient do feel more confident and able to manage the stresses arising from the giving of care. Thus it is necessary for staff to attend conferences and workshops which are now being provided through hospice education centres and organizations such as Help the Hospices, the Marie Curie Foundation and Cancer Relief.

It must not be thought that these activities are designed only for the needs of health professionals. There are many others who are also involved in the care of the dying, such as clergy, pastoral care assistants and volunteers. Most clergy would agree that their theological college training sent them out ill-equipped to handle the more acute aspects of pastoral care as identified in a study by Murray (1990) among Scottish clergy. Much cannot be taught in theoretical isolation, but much has to be faced, very often alone, by the minister when once ordained. The provision of ongoing training and support is therefore vital and is today being provided through a number of channels.

Pastoral teamwork must never be overlooked as it is possibly the most valuable resource available. Everyone involved in this work, continually feeling their own inadequacy, can be drained and saturated by the environment of loss to the point that sensitivity and the capacity to give are diminished to near uselessness. To be able to offload and share with others is of the utmost help.

REFERENCES

Braun, P.J. and Katz, L.F. (1989) A study of burnout in nurses working in hospice and hospital oncology settings. *Oncology Nursing Forum*, **16**(4), 18–20.

Eakes, C.G. (1990) Grief resolution in hospice nurses. *Nursing and Health Care*, **11**(5), 243–8.

Farrell, M. (1992) A process of mutual support. *Professional Nurse*, **7**(3), 10–12, 14.

Fisher, M. (1991) Can grief be turned into growth? *Professional Nurse*, **7**(3), 178–82.

Harris, L. (1988) Breaking bad news. Communicating with the dying patient and family. *Nursing Times*, **84** (suppl.), Community Outlook, (19) 15–17.

McKerrow, L. (1991) Dealing with stress of caring for the dying in intensive care unit: an overview. *Intensive Care Nursing*, **7**(4), 219–22.

Murray, D.B. (1990) The education and training of Scottish clergy in the care of the dying. *Palliative Medicine*, **4**(1), 18.

Neuberger, J. (1986) A crying shame. *Nursing Times*, **82**, 22.

Owen, G. (1991) Do you give your staff support? *THS Health Summary*, **8**(3), 14.

Penson, J. (1990) *Bereavement – A Guide for Nurses*, Harper and Row, London, p. 162.

Quoist, M. (1968) *The Christian Response*, Gill and Son, Dublin, p. 51.

Scott, G. (1993) The RCN Cancer Nursing Society Annual Conference. *Nursing Standard*, **7**(39), 15.

Stoller, E. P. (1988) Effect of experience on nurses' responses to dying and death in a hospital setting. *Nursing Research*, (1988) Vol. 29. No. 1. p. 35.

13 Religious beliefs and cultural issues

THE SPIRITUAL DIMENSION

Pastoral care is based on the existence of God (whatever be His name) and the spiritual dimension of humanity. It is an anthropological fact that humanity, by its very nature, is prone towards a divinity, towards a god; this can also be seen from basic everyday observation. This tendency can be found in humanity in whatever age and set of circumstances; it is a common observation right across the spectrum of humankind. If this is true and if our total patient care is to be really 'total', then we must face up to and 'nurse' the spiritual dimension of the patient.

There are particular times in life when these concepts take on a special urgency – times of joy and sorrow, times of danger and risk. Among these occasions, periods of sickness and, of course, terminal illness bring us face to face with destiny, with inevitability, with the unknown. There does not seem to be a choice in this. Even though our Western culture has 'successfully' marginalized death and dying out of sight, all of this enlightenment can come crashing down as the patient (and relatives too) comes face to face with the inevitability of imminent personal death. For better or worse the patient grapples with the meaning of humanity, the meaning of life and death and the possibility of life hereafter; all take on, in a new and very personal way, a significance that is both immediate and relevant. Death as a phenomenon or indeed as a reality for other people now becomes very personal and has to be approached in a very personal way. Death is not just at **a** doorstep, it is at **my** doorstep. Such a realization causes the mind to concentrate.

At this stage we are at the heart of the spiritual dimension and the chaplain is part of it. It is for the chaplain (as part of the overall caring team) to stay with the patient, the all-important person whose past is over, whose present is limited in time and whose future is filled with a newness never experienced before. At this stage, thoughts of the past –

guilt feelings, regrets, bad self-image – can crowd the mind. Is this a punishment, an abandonment by God? This is the situation into which the chaplain arrives.

The confrontation with death has but one outcome. Caring for the spiritual dimension means helping the patient to confront death with life-giving hope rather than with life-destroying fear. The emphasis is on the precious gift of life; the patient is living in a terminal state, not dying with it. Conscious of their own struggles with the mysteries of life and death and with the mystery of God, chaplains are both a symbol of strength and at the same time a witness to finality and helplessness. While it may be true that they have come to grips with their own faith and through faith, answers to the problems of life, they cannot presume that faith can guarantee the answers to another's problems. Experience shows that with faith it is indeed possible to face up to death and all its implications, but this may be stated more in hindsight than a priori in the case of any individual person.

The experience over the years of dealing with the challenges of life and of faith can also contribute greatly to a balanced and positive approach to death. However, this constructive approach is not confined only to those who have had a successful and balanced life. Chaplains everywhere (and carers too) continually meet up with patients who, without any experience of religious practice, have a resilience and an inner strength where none would have been anticipated. The spiritual dimension is one area that does not permit generalization. Caring for the spiritual dimension can open the way to a patient's discovery of a personal God. The pace of their own discovery is unique to every individual. True caring recognizes this individuality and treats it with the maximum respect and encouragement.

THE CHRISTIAN RELIGION

All Christians have a common belief in the meaning of the death and resurrection of Jesus Christ. For the Christian, Jesus came that we may have life and have it to the full (*John* 10:10). Death contains within itself the moment of resurrection and it was for that rebirth that Christ came on earth. His death, leading to His resurrection, gives meaning to our life and also to our death. 'We believe that having died with Christ we shall return to life with him' (Romans 6:8). This clear and resounding statement is the core of the Christian declaration about death. Well tested over the centuries, it continues to provide solid comfort to the dying.

For the Christian, the dead are no longer dead but living in Christ. Death therefore is seen in the context of life. It is part of both this life and life hereafter. It belongs to life as an end and a beginning. It is rightly called a rebirth. This is the Christian attitude to death: 'Life is changed, not ended' (Requiem Mass). It is the moment of liberation. The only ending is an ending of exile and of human limitation.

The Christian chaplain is there to be available to any who wish to 'talk things over'. When the comment is made that it is good to have someone there for that purpose, it is a sign of reassurance and relief that the patient feels the support and back-up from another human being who declares gently the normality of sickness and death. What is beautifully human is already a step into the spiritual. The chaplain's easy pace and presence can in itself be a witness to the patient of a living and caring God. Patients need such an opening and experience shows that in their own time and in the uniqueness of their individuality, the spiritual dimension is brought to the surface.

Pastoral care of the family

It is rare that a patient has neither family, relatives nor friends. Total patient care cannot overlook caring for the unique and intimate relationship between the patient and those accompanying them at the end of their life. With impending separation and loss, these special people have special needs at that time. Pastoral care, with its central message of salvation, should accompany the family members in their efforts to cope in this highly charged emotional time of their lives. The central message to the patient is also the message to the family, relatives and friends. What is positive for one is positive for all.

Sometimes chaplains will find a far greater challenge from the family, whose helplessness and anger are often placed on God. They may therefore encounter rebuff and even hostility. In these situations, chaplains should be able to accept such reaction, knowing that it is not meant personally. At times like this the personal encounter with a key member of the family can be greatly beneficial. Seeing the patient as a member of the family, the care of the patient and that of the family can be mutually supportive and sustaining.

The hospice with its particular facilities can also provide the immediate family and all the relatives and friends with an image of the spiritual dimension that is the basis of pastoral care. The best guideline is the individual attention and appreciation of every person involved in the patient's illness and death. This is further enhanced by the caring hospice atmosphere provided by the ambience and all the staff.

Promoting spiritual awareness in the staff

Very often members of the staff find themselves at a loss when it comes to the spiritual needs of their patients. The easy way out is to promise to call the chaplain, whose 'speciality' is in that sphere. This indicates uncertainty rather than unwillingness to become involved.

It is up to the chaplain to highlight the valuable part that staff members can play by simply staying with the patient as a listening and reassuring friend. After all, it was the patient who, in the first place, chose that particular member of the staff with whom to share. Moreover, members of the staff need to be aware that they, and not the chaplain, may be chosen by the patient as being easier to share with in matters spiritual than the official (and professional) minister of religion. Tradition, ignorance, prejudice, superstition and previous bad experience can create barriers that make an encounter with the chaplain appear threatening, especially at the initial stage. It is essential for chaplains themselves to experience the support of the staff and to foster the staff's participation with them in the spiritual care of the patient.

Care of the bereaved

Bereavement work is a complex and prolonged ministry. It, too, can be helped by the spiritual care given before the death and after. The Christian assurances to the patient remain the spiritual background on which the pastoral care of the bereaved is based. The funeral rites are an important stage in the bereavement process and should therefore be given careful attention by the chaplain. An intimate and deeply personal funeral service can set the tone for the beginning of recovery from grief and loss and is, for the chaplain, a privileged moment of care for the bereaved. Since it is a once-only and a group event, it should be conducted with the utmost sensitivity and simplicity. The understanding of the rites may be hindered for the mourners by the emotional upheaval they are experiencing. Much good can be achieved at funeral services. The opposite can also be true.

ROMAN CATHOLIC MINISTRY

Apart from private prayer with the individual patient (and when appropriate with the family) the Roman Catholic ministry to the sick is made up of the liturgical celebration of the sacraments: the Eucharist, the Sacrament of the Sick (the Anointing) and the Sacrament of Reconciliation (previously called Confession).

Personal prayer ought to be simple, taking into account the limited energy of the patient. Short Bible readings and traditional prayers read or recited slowly can also be very helpful. Account must be taken of those who have lost contact with any formal prayer. Above all there should be no crowding of the patient with long and drawn out prayers.

The sacraments are ideally celebrated in a community setting. At home this might be with members of the family, friends and neighbours, some perhaps from the local church. In a hospital or hospice it may be possible to gather several Roman Catholics in the chapel or some other small room to celebrate together. Again, any relatives, friends or staff members would ideally form a community. It has also been found in a hospice setting that non-Catholic patients are happy to be present at the Eucharistic celebration and feel a bond with their Catholic fellow patients. Equally the chaplain will be happy to bring the sacraments to an individual Catholic patient in private. Readings should be chosen with care; direct reference to the topic of death or dying should be avoided in group sharing since the chaplain has no control over the resulting impact on individual patients.

The Sacrament of Reconciliation is a powerful means of restoring a positive self-image and self-confidence to the patient. Extreme sensitivity is needed on the part of the chaplain whose patients may have strong feelings of guilt and negative past experiences. Care must also be taken to allow the patient true freedom in choosing the appropriate moment to celebrate this sacrament. It is not uncommon to find a patient pressurized by family members who wish them to 'make their peace with God'.

The Sacrament of the Sick has recovered its original meaning and purpose. Until relatively recently it was known as the Last Rites or Extreme Unction and was generally administered in association with imminent death. There may be still some patients whose images of this sacrament remains the same as that of their parents' or grandparents' time. The sacrament is best celebrated during the celebration of the Eucharist and, if possible, in the company of family and staff members.

THE ANGLICAN MINISTRY

Experience and the present-day scene both suggest that the traditional Church of England approach, which assumed a familiarity with the accepted forms of communication and liturgy, must now be sensitively reconsidered.

Pastoral care of the dying, the despairing and the bereaved must, above all, seek to reach each individual at the present point of their experience with the reassuring security of God and in a way they can understand.

For those who are regular worshippers in an Anglican setting there is a ready resource of hope-inspiring scripture and relevant prayers to be found in the *Book of Common Prayer*, the *Alternative Service Book* and the booklet *Ministry to the Sick*. For the troubled at heart an opportunity for simple confession to God, accompanied by a positive affirmation of forgiveness on the basis of the death of Christ, may bring untold relief.

The ministry of Anointing has deeply Biblical roots and may with sensitivity bring a sense of healing and wholeness of the inner being in time of great crisis. For the believer a simple presentation of Holy Communion brings into clear focus the deeply personal impact of the sacrifice and resurrection of Christ.

Too often nobody thinks of informing the clergy, yet they are expected to know what is happening! Consultation between carers will help establish the level and form the support should take. Usually the minister will bring all that is needed for a service at the bedside, but whether in hospital or at home it is important that the setting allows for personal preparation of mind and for the occasion to be received meaningfully. A period of quietness beforehand; a small table by the bedside simply set with a white cloth and flowers; a general air of calm and supportive warmth; these all help to prepare patient and family to receive strength and reassurance through worship and the word of God.

These are traditional paths but the chaplain and the nurse will find increasingly that they are unfamiliar to many they are called to care for. Religious practice may be so remote from such people that it can not offer sufficient relevance to help them and the set prayers from a book may serve only to increase their sense of distance and isolation. Here the immediacy of the held hand and the burden-sharing reality of simple, open and honest listening which slips naturally into prayer may provide the most helpful way for the sufferer to discover the surrounding protection of God.

Care for the patient must never preclude the family's needs. A whole range of largely unspoken emotions may lie beneath the surface. The nurse or minister may be the one to help bring together broken relationships; to resolve the deceptions often practised in the name of love, yet which can leave the patient feeling isolated from nearest and dearest; to convey to the household the recognition that goodbye must be said and to give the confidence to be able to say it. Where the family is sensitively led through these stages it will help the patient to leave peacefully and the family to be able to look back upon a departure that has not left them with loose ends that can never be resolved.

In this connection it is important too to be alert to children and to the emotional damage that can result from their exclusion. They are as much part of the family as a limb is part of a body and too many children have grown up carrying anger and resentment over the way they were shut out from family illness and death. With insight and love the carer may be able to do what the family cannot cope with, explaining the illness and prognosis in very simple terms, allowing the child to say goodbye and explaining the significance of the funeral so that the child can decide whether or not to attend. Later the whole experience becomes a matter for the entire family to share and work through together.

The importance of telling a child the truth cannot be overemphasized and as Christians we have ample resources to be able to explain. Damage can be done through resorting to fairytale ideas or insensitive clichés which can give a false idea of the God we want the child to trust in.

The family may well appreciate guidance over the funeral, in particular where there may be little active link with a church. The minister should be as well acquainted as possible both with the deceased, so as to be able to speak honestly, and with the family so as to be able to pray for them realistically. The options of a service in church or crematorium should be discussed and whether the deceased wished burial or cremation and, in the latter case, how to dispose of the ashes in a manner helpful to the family. There can be considerable scope in making a funeral service personal and for it to be a memorable occasion which will help greatly in the process of healing. Hymns and readings chosen by the family and the relaxed and personal use of their names during the service bring a lift to proceedings. The presence of nurses or doctor at a funeral will always be an encouragement and may even be, for them, a necessary stage in letting go.

For any carer, nurse or chaplain, perhaps the greatest asset is to recognize that the religious contrivances of the familiar church scene are no more than the optional tools, of greatly varying usefulness, provided from a long tradition of distilled experience. What will ultimately be of greatest help to the sufferer will be the realization of their own worth and of their acceptance by a God of love. Our job is to effect the introduction. This is no more the role of the religious professional than it is of the nurse who, with one hand in the hand of God, cares enough to reach out with the other and become at that moment the Holy Spirit's channel to bring forgiveness, peace, assurance and hope.

Spiritual ministry should therefore not be seen as some religious appendage to the programme of palliative care, but as a vital and integral contribution to the sense of wholeness for both patient and family. A sense of spiritual well-being enhances quality of life for the patient and brings healing into the ongoing experience of the family. The ordeal of terminal illness inflicts disintegration upon a household, bringing stress into relationships, destroying self-confidence and diminishing self-worth, fragmenting hope and churning up new and deep emotions. It is care for the spiritual dimension above all which can, when accepted, help to reorder and strengthen what is being violently pulled apart.

Everyone in the arena of offering spiritual care feels the need for backup. Sometimes our tank runs dry and we need to draw upon another's resources, knowing that our client will be better helped. Whether in hospice, hospital or in the community the carer's greatest resource is carers. We should allow a network of mutual trust to interweave and draw together the availability of skilled and sensitive Christians, so that in any given district resources from across the professions are immediately available, clergy, nurses, social workers, doctors, each with their special insights and all with a Godgiven sense of responsibility to offer His love in a way that makes it as easy as possible to accept.

FREE CHURCHES

These Christian Churches make up the third group of mainstream churches in the UK and share with the Anglican and Roman Catholics a belief in the Trinity, the assurance of eternal life and the *Holy Bible*.

Both patients and their families will receive spiritual help and comfort from the prayers of their families and fellow Christians.

There are few, if any, rites in relation to the dying patient, although the sacrament of Holy Communion plays a very important part in the life of many Free Church adherents. For a minister, relative or friend just to sit with a patient quietly, perhaps just holding hands and listening, is always a great comfort.

Free Church chaplains come under the umbrella of the Free Church Federal Council, who amongst many other activities have a Hospital Chaplaincy Board responsible for the training and appointment of hospice and hospital chaplains.

The Free Church Federal Council is made up of about 15 separate independent churches, the largest of which are the Methodist Church, the Baptist Church, the United Reformed Church and the Salvation Army. In addition to this organization, their chaplains are often members of the College of Health Care Chaplains or the Association of Hospice Chaplains, both of which are ecumenical groups and aim to maintain standards of excellence with their members.

NON-CHRISTIAN RELIGIOUS FAITHS

Anyone caring for a dying patient in Britain today will certainly meet a proportion of people from a totally different religious background than the traditional Christian society (however nominal in practice) which used to include the majority of the population. Now a hospital ward may include patients of several of the main non-Christian faiths, with all shades of orthodoxy. There are also people who have no specific religion or religious and cultural tradition which might give them comfort and help in the last days, weeks or months of life. Among this group, some will be firm in their attitude that they neither need nor wish for any religious ministrations, describing themselves as humanists. This should, of course, be respected.

Responsibilities of the nurse and other carers

Nurses in particular have an important role in recognizing how valuable it is for the dying patient's comfort to respond to the practical aspects of their religious faith. In Chapter 6, detailed guidelines are given on caring for patients of the following world religions:

- Judaism
- Sikhism
- Hinduism
- Islam
- Buddhism.

Attention to practical needs will be enhanced if the nurse has made an effort to learn something of the background beliefs of the particular faith and the culture with which they are associated, so that when first meeting the patient they have the sense of interest and the wish to be helpful. It is not always easy, as there are many other religions and sects whose adherents may enter hospital or hospice when dying and information may not be immediately available, especially if there are language barriers. Consulting the family is obviously the first resource after the patient and clear concise guidelines should be available in patient areas, including telephone numbers of religious centres where further information could be obtained.

Understanding a little more leads ideally to respect and compassion. 'Suddenly, here is someone who knows what might be required, who has taken the trouble to find out something about the individual patient's religion and culture and who is offering to make special provision for the individual' (Neuberger, 1987).

REFERENCES

Neuberger, J. (1987) *Caring for Dying People of Different Faiths*, Lisa Sainsbury Foundation Series, Austen Cornish, London.

FURTHER READING

Cassidy, S. (1988) *Sharing the Darkness*, Darton, Longman and Todd, London.

Lothian Community Relations Council (1984) *Religious Cultures*, LCRC, Edinburgh.

McGilloway, O. and Myco, F. (eds) (1985) *Nursing and Spiritual Care*, Harper and Row, London.

Sampson, C. (1982) *The Neglected Ethic*, McGraw-Hill, Maidenhead.

Speck, P. (1988) *Being There*, SPCK, London.
Twycross, R. (ed.) (1991) *Mud and Stars*, Sobell Publications, Oxford.
Walker, C. (1982) Attitudes to death and bereavement among cultural minority groups. *Nursing Times*, **78**(50), 2106–9.

14 Ethical aspects

> Ethics is not a subject to be left in the hands of academics. It is a subject which needs to be used and understood by the staff working with patients. These are the people who are involved in making these difficult decisions.
>
> (Crump, 1990)

Even within the last few years, new and disturbing questions of an ethical nature seem to challenge those responsible for the provision of health care in an ever-increasing stream. The dramatic advances in science and medical technology threaten to outstrip the traditional body of information and knowledge on ethical considerations, yet doctors in particular are expected to give instant answers to difficult questions in the full glare of the media. It is of course right that society should take an intense interest in ethical question and it is increasingly recognized that patients and their relations should be brought into the consultation process for decisions of great personal importance.

Other health care professionals must also take responsibility for their own evolving ethnical codes of practice. Nursing ethics is not simply a reflection of medical ethics, although of course closely linked with these, since nurses have many unique responsibilities towards patients. Hospital managers in the changing National Health Service have a heavy responsibility in the ethical use of resources.

In the context of this book, consideration of ethics in health care must be confined to issues relating to the end of human life which have particular contemporary urgency for health care practitioners in palliative care.

EUTHANASIA

In June 1993 Dr Stuart Horner, Chairman of the British Medical Association's ethical committee, said that euthanasia is neither more nor less than the murder of patients and should have no place in the practice of medicine. The conference at which he spoke declared by a majority of about 5:1 that it 'categorically rejected' legalization of euthanasia in a debate following the recent case of Dr Nigel Cox, a rheumatologist found guilty of the attempted murder of an elderly patient dying in pain.

This clear and unambiguous viewpoint is not, of course, shared by all doctors and nurses, although probably by the majority and by those of the general public who are well informed about the implications of euthanasia were it to be legalized. In no country has a legal right been established for a deliberately hastened death. Yet in the Netherlands, although euthanasia is prohibited in law, it is protected by both lower and supreme court decisions and is thus effectively tolerated legally. There are disturbing statistics about actual practice where problems of unconscious and incompetent patients are not covered by existing Dutch guidelines – and also that adequate palliative care is not always offered or available (Gomez, 1991).

This last point is a crucial one for those in our own country who are demonstrating by their practice of excellence in care of dying patients in hospital, hospice or at home, that it is possible to control to a considerable degree distressing symptoms, especially pain, and enable patients to die peacefully and comfortably. This is the answer to the protagonists of euthanasia – unfortunately, it is still not the situation everywhere in the United Kingdom, let alone in the Netherlands.

SELECTIVE NON-TREATMENT

This is sometimes described as passive euthanasia but considered by some to be better described under the alternative heading. However, this is arguable (Rachels, 1975).

There is a moral obligation to the terminally ill, as to any other patient, to provide basic physical care. This includes giving food and water by mouth as long as the patient is able to take it. This duty to a patient of any age was legally upheld in 1981 in the case of a doctor (Leonard Arthur) who gave instructions for 'nursing care only' in a physically healthy Down's syndrome baby whose parents did not wish it to survive. A criminal prosecution was brought against the doctor. One has great sympathy for the nurses involved in this situation. 'Nursing care' has always included feeding patients and providing fluids.

A very difficult issue is when artificial feeding is the only possible means of nutrition and fluid intake and the possible benefit of continuing this indefinitely is in question. This dilemma was dramatically highlighted in 1993 in the case of Tony Bland, aged 22 years. A victim of the Hillsborough football disaster, he had been in an irreversible coma for four years. After full consultation with all concerned (and at the request of his parents) his nasogastric tube was removed and thus feeding and hydration ceased. Tony died ten days later. The case aroused a storm of debate regarding the morality of the decision, illustrating how complex the issue is. On the one hand, it was argued that feeding and giving fluid are not medical treatments but a basic duty of care. On the other hand many would argue that tube feeding is an artificial method and may be compared to the artificial maintenance of breathing by a ventilator. In the latter case, it is generally held to be morally justifiable to turn off the ventilator or indeed to terminate any medical treatment when that can no longer be designated as therapeutic. The case of Tony Bland was given further significance by the legal ruling of the Law Lords that the cessation of tube feeding was permissible in this case as 'his life was now futile' and thus the patient's doctor was not at risk of prosecution for murder. There was a general consensus of opinion among those who did not condemn the decision absolutely that the decision was based on a false argument and that great vigilance is needed if a general slide towards euthanasia is not to happen. It should be noted that there are over 1000 other patients in the UK in the so-called persistent vegetative state similar to Tony Bland.

> It has been argued that pictures of starvation and dehydration as witnessed on television from 3rd world countries do not apply to the process in a dying patient, the aged and those with severe neurological impairments. Such patients may not be technically unconscious but neither are they 'alert'. Deprivation of fluid rapidly results in further depression of consciousness and ultimately coma. There is some evidence for impaired sensation of thirst in these circumstances and for endogenous production of substances producing natural analgesia.
> (Ahronheim and Gasner, 1990)

> Tube feeding itself may produce pain from erosion of the nasal septum or haemorrhage from oesophagus and gastric mucosa. Until recently, people who grew very old, too weak or too ill to eat died without a feeding tube in place. It may be assumed that rejection of food is a physiological component of grave illness and of dying. Harrowing pictures of a cruel and violent death do not seem to be borne out by observers who have witnessed peaceful death in the comatose patient.
> (Ahronheim and Gasner, 1990)

The above observations do not directly answer the question as to whether cessation of tube feeding is always morally justifiable, but might support the proposition that the burdens involved for the patient and their family may be considered so great as to outweigh the benefits of prolonging life by artificial means. However, the decision has to be founded on medical grounds, i.e. how far the treatment itself can still be termed therapeutic.

The actual practice of tube feeding is carried out by nurses in most instances. It is thus essential that they should be involved throughout in any decisions to be made regarding the continuation or cessation of the regime.

> In the end, it seems possible only to lay down the minimum requirement which is that nutrition and hydration should never be withheld from a patient who is able to take them normally by mouth. No argument as to the quality of life should be allowed to obscure this basic principle of humanity.
>
> (Mason, 1988)

There are, of course, other areas of selective non-treatment which are commonly practised and require consideration of the ethical issues involved.

CARE OF THE TERMINALLY ILL PATIENT

In palliative medicine there may be a number of occasions when, having weighed up the benefits and burdens of a proposed course of action, the doctor may decide, for instance:

- not to prescribe an antibiotic for the terminally ill patient with pneumonia;
- not to give a blood transfusion to a patient whose dying is complicated by bleeding from the upper or lower gastrointestinal tract.

What could be done is not necessarily what should be done. 'The prolongation of life should not itself constitute the exclusive aim of medical practice, which must be concerned equally with the relief of suffering' (Council of Europe, 1976).

A patient has a right to refuse treatment and to have their choice respected, as long as they are lucid and capable of understanding the issues involved. When this is not the case, the patient's family and nursing staff, as well as the physician in charge, should all be involved in decisions not to initiate or prolong active treatment. This is not a negative attitude of abdicating responsibility for the patient's well-being, but the time for expanding much effort in controlling distressing symptoms without extraordinary and sophisticated measures.

USE OF POWERFUL OPIATE OR SEDATIVE DRUGS

Relief of pain and distress is an important responsibility of both doctors and nurses towards patients. In the case of the dying patient, administration of drugs as part of the treatment should be uncontroversial where a proper regime is used, as described in Chapter 6. The question as to whether it is ethical to administer large doses of drugs at the possible expense of shortening the patient's life has been fully explored and an answer given which is generally accepted. It is based on the principle known as 'double effect', widely accepted in Christian theology, whereby a good action is not forbidden even if one of its unintended consequences is evil. In practice, with skilled pain control, pain-killing drugs such as morphine are thought to have little effect on life expectancy (Mason, 1988). An anxiety is sometimes expressed that a nurse does not wish to be the one to give 'the last injection', implying that it is this that will end the patient's life. This is erroneous; the patient having pain control management as described in Chapter 6 dies from the disease, not from the drug administered.

The opposite situation may occur where the nurse considers that a patient is receiving inadequate analgesia and is in pain, but the doctor appears to be reluctant to alter the medication. Consulting with an experienced nursing colleague and then both discussing the matter with the doctor are the appropriate steps to take to resolve the problem.

ADAVANCE DIRECTIVES/LIVING WILLS

There is a good deal of current interest in these documents and their use is widespread in the USA. An advance directive is a statement made by a fully competent person about the health care they would wish to receive if they became incompetent. A 'living will' is usually taken to be a special type of advance directive concerned with refusing life-prolonging treatment (Hope, 1992).

Those documents are encouraged by the Voluntary Euthanasia Society, who have drawn up such directives. Malcolm Harwith (Chairman) is open about the fact that he sees them as a stop-gap on the way to voluntary euthanasia 'but any legislation for advance directives or voluntary euthanasia must always contain a conscience clause for doctors and nurses who do not want to be involved'.

Both the RCN and BMA advise caution about treating advance directives as anything other than one factor to be taken into account when difficult clinical decisions have to be taken. Although the patient's written wishes should be treated with the utmost respect, people may change their mind over a period of years and then may no longer be able to communicate this easily.

ORGAN DONATION

Respect for the body of a deceased person is a feature of all religious and secular belief systems. Although this involves different practices in various cultures, for the most part violation of the body's integrity for transplantation because of its humanitarian aspect is mainly acceptable. This includes Jewish society and, in principle, Islamic countries. In Japan, there is a barrier to acceptance of a brain-related concept of death since in traditional Japanese thought it is the gut which symbolically represents the major organs.

There are potential ethical dilemmas in the removal of organs. The main source of supply is in the intensive therapy unit from patients who have been ventilated. Sometimes, patients dying from cerebrovascular accident in a general ward may have an elective ventilation for the purpose of organ donations. This poses a distressing situation for relatives and nurses.

More recently patients dying from terminal cancer at St Christopher's Hospice have donated kidneys and heart valves – this appears to give comfort to their relatives. There are, of course, contraindications, but the outcome for recipients has been quite encouraging. Corneal donation has been common for many years in a number of hospices.

There are many ethical questions surrounding organ transplants. Firstly, in the case of living donors it must be ensured that consent is freely given and that the risk is not too great. The motivation must not be one of suicidal or homicidal intent, out of financial desperation or, in the case of prisoners, in the expectation of custodial relief. In recent years there have been a number of scandals in Europe and the USA involving trafficking in human organs for financial gain. The need for transplantable organs is greater than the supply, especially for kidneys. In the UK there are heart-rending reports of approximately 4000 people on dialysis awaiting surgery. Added to this are those awaiting heart, lung and liver transplants. The government supports campaigns to encourage people to put down in writing their wish to donate organs after their death. Consideration is also being given for an alternative scheme – that a dead person's organs can be used automatically if no statement of a contrary nature has been made whilst they were alive. In other words, consent is presumed. The urgency of the quest for donors highlights another example of the marvels of medical technology and subsequent success in saving lives creating its own ethical problems.

There are two major issues of disquiet among the general public which have to be allayed:

1. In the case of cadaveric donors, is the donor really dead at the time of removal of organs? 'It would be preferable by far for man's future survival to have to abandon transplantation than to agree to remove vital organs from individuals who are not really dead' (Report of the Conference of European Health Ministers, 1987).
2. How can the duty of care to the potential donor up to the point of

death, and the instinctive respect for the integrity of the human body even when no longer a living person, be balanced with the duty of efforts to save the life of a person with a life-threatening condition? These are daunting problems, especially for staff working in operating theatres and intensive therapy units. The background to the issues is to define what is understood by 'death'.

The majority of British doctors are content with the concept of brainstem death and after specific tests for this accuracy, removal of organs will be permitted from the dead donor who is being ventilated.

> Official recognition of brain death came in two stages in the United Kingdom. In the first, the conference of the Medical Royal Colleges and their faculties (1976) – certainly the greatest concentration of medical expertise available – laid down the diagnostic criteria which consisted, primarily, of the often forgotten conditions for considering the diagnosis of brain death and, then, of specific tests for establishing its occurrence. In the second phase (1979) it was agreed that the identification of brainstem death means that the patient is dead, whether or not the functions of some organs, such as a heartbeat, are still maintained by artificial means.
>
> (Mason, 1988)

To avoid potential conflicts between the attending physician and the needs of the transplant team, it is ensured that the donor's physician should not have a role in the transplantation procedure itself. Although the ethical problem may have been solved to the satisfaction of most people involved, it cannot but be a matter of emotional recoil for most people that since kidneys must be perfused *in situ* within the donor patient's body until immediately after the organ retrieval surgery, this means the presence of a heartbeat whilst the organs are removed. One must reiterate that there should be awareness of the strain on relatives whilst all this is going on and for the nursing staff and rest of the professional team.

SUICIDE

This must be one of the most distressing forms of dying and death, both for the individual and their family. The majority of suicides are carried out by people who are suffering from severe clinical depression and thus in a disturbed frame of mind. Feelings of loneliness and despair may be impossible to share and about one third of those who take their own lives give no warning of their intention. For the relatives, there are always agonizing questions: Why did it happen? What could I have done to prevent it? Where the person contemplating suicide gives some sign of this, anyone whose sympathetic support is acceptable – whether family, friends or caring staff of the individual if in hospital – may be able to avert a catastrophe, for the time being at any rate. In 1953 Chad Varah founded The Samaritans in response to the suicide of a young girl, with the aim of providing a 24-hour listening (telephone) service for those who were suicidal. In 1992 about 2.5 million calls of this nature were answered.

A doctor may find themselves in a difficult moral and legal situation (as may a nurse) if confronted by a patient who has attempted suicide but is still alive. A competent person is entitled to refuse treatment for a lethal condition and this includes a primary suicide attempt. So a doctor risks being prosecuted for assault if, for instance, they initiate gastric lavage against the expressed wish of the patient. In practice, the legal response is likely to be favourable since the doctor may reasonably assume that the patient is not competent to make a rational choice due to a disturbed state of mind.

If a doctor or a nurse works in the prison health service, they may be involved with prisoners who have undertaken hunger strikes, usually for political reasons. This is of course a form of suicide. Again, it must be an intolerable situation for those who wish to offer medical or nursing help to stand aside, which they must do. Once near to death, force feeding is permissible in the United Kingdom if considered to be beneficial. The 1961 Suicide Act removes suicide from the list of criminal offences. However, aiding and abetting a suicide remains a serious criminal offence.

RESUSCITATION AND USE OF LIFE-SUPPORT SYSTEMS

In a general hospital it may be a student nurse who initiates resuscitation in a patient who suddenly suffers cardiac arrest. Clear guidance is essential in the ward as to when this procedure should be carried out and for which patients it is inappropriate. The staff should understand why particular decisions are made. Good communications will remove uncertainty and worry that the 'wrong' action has been taken or not. Nurses will be very involved in the care of a patient whose vital functions are being maintained by a life-support system. If it is thought to be no longer reasonable to continue ventilation of the patient because brainstem death has been confirmed, the medical staff in charge should discuss the matter with the family and with the whole caring team before the machine is switched off. This is a traumatic situation for all concerned and it should be made clear that this is not a case of killing the patient, because they are already dead.

Cardiopulmonary resuscitation is particularly difficult in a ward situation, being inevitably a public crisis which must temporarily disrupt nursing care of other patients. Afterwards if the resuscitation attempt has been unsuccessful, there must be comfort and support of grieving relatives and frightened patients as well as the emotionally stressed staff. The decision 'not to resuscitate' remains the exception in hospital, usually on the authority of the medical consultant or senior registrar.

BASIC PRINCIPLES

Ethics is the study of morals – that is, the distinction between right and wrong behaviour. The classical Christian approach to general ethical questions has been through the concept of Natural Law. It is assumed to be possible, in the light of reason and divine revelation, to discern the laws by which human beings should live, i.e. that there are fundamental moral principles based on the dignity of the human person and their basic rights which are universal at all times.

So far as medicine is concerned, any deliberate interference with normal bodily functioning is, according to this view, a violation of Natural Law but may be justified on one of two main principles:

1. the 'principle of totality' whereby any diseased part of the body may be removed or otherwise modified if its malfunctioning constitutes a serious threat to the whole;
2. the principle of 'double effect' already described earlier in this chapter.

(Dunstan and Dunstan, 1981)

Ethical principles, however, are formulated to guide in decisions about concrete problems and needs. Their development is influenced by current knowledge, cultural environment and religious beliefs. In the specific field of palliative care or of sudden life-threatening situations, a nurse or doctor often has to act under great pressure and make quick decisions. It is therefore important to have thought about one's own attitudes and to search one's conscience. This is a duty to oneself, to patients and to colleagues.

For instance, a nurse may be working in an operating theatre and suddenly refuses on moral grounds to assist the surgeon who is performing an abortion. If the patient starts to bleed heavily, the nurse would be held gravely at fault if they did not remain during this crisis and give assistance to save the patient's life. The law in this country provides a dissociation clause for non-participation in abortion and the nurse should have made their position clear to the theatre superintendent well in advance.

A good deal of anxiety is currently expressed about an apparent shift from the traditional sanctity of life ethos to a quality of life position which is reflected in professional ethics, especially among doctors and nurses. This is taking place in a pluralistic and largely agnostic society (Mason, 1988). The powerful influence of professional attitudes among the general population and the emergence of 'situation ethics' or the 'feel-good factor' is prevalent, especially among young people. However, Clifford Longley (1993) thinks that the ethical framework towards which young people are searching and their intuitive moral insights should not be dismissed too readily, being akin to the traditional view of conscience as an inner voice of moral guidance.

The dangers of the 'slippery slope' slide towards moral anarchy do appear to present ever-increasing challenges to our present society, increasing the burdens of those engaged in health care. Twycross (1990) warns doctors considering whether becoming involved in physician-assisted death might be justifiable in some circumstances that, in his belief, 'it would be a disaster for the medical profession to cross the Rubicon'. He reminds his readers of the situation in abortion which is now performed on demand in considerable numbers year after year, which was not at all the intention of those who enabled the act of 1967 to be passed. That is, what begins as an occasional practice within strict limits tends to lead to a massive increase eventually.

THE DYING PATIENT – APPLYING ETHICAL PRINCIPLES IN ACTUAL SITUATIONS

1. Where the patient is conscious and competent to make decisions, they have the right to be consulted where there is a choice between continuing active treatment or not. For instance, a question of further radiotherapy may arise in advancing cancer, which the patient has a right to refuse. The patient's family should be involved and all appropriate members of the caring team.
2. Where the patient is not competent and decisions have to be made, those caring for them must ask themselves:
   - What is in the best interests of this individual?
   - What would the individual choose for themselves if they were able to do so?
   - What is considered to be the right moral choice?

   These considerations would apply to children and the mentally handicapped, as well as unconscious adults.
3. When the needs of a group of patients have to be considered in life or death situations, the questions of priority in allocating scarce resources can pose acute ethical dilemmas. It may be in choosing which desperately ill patient should be offered a heart transplant or dialysis machine. Can neonatal intensive care units cope with rising numbers of very premature infants who are likely to die unless admitted to such units? In the fearful situation of recent civil wars in several countries, where hospitals are without even basic resources to treat casualties, even starker choices have to be made in attempting to save lives.

It is here that professional experience, common sense and one's own informed conscience regarding moral principles are so important. The situation is often very difficult and doctors and nurses are fallible human beings, however experienced.

It may happen that two professional people have differing though sincerely held views about a decision and subsequent action involving a moral choice. It is commendable to have the courage of one's convictions and to state them. If a nurse was concerned about their involvement in a situation where a doctor was treating a patient, e.g. they are asked to administer a drug and do not consider it right to do so, then they are entitled to refuse. However, it is obviously advisable to make sure that they are in full possession of the facts and not jumping to the wrong conclusion. Refusal to cooperate is a serious matter.

It is encouraging that many hospitals and community care authorities have set up ethical committees to provide venues for discussion and informed debate about the increasing number of ethical problems posed by modern medicine and scientific advances. Ethical issues are frequent subjects for articles and letters in professional journals, as well as in the daily newspapers.

CONCLUSION

To end on a personal note; having presented various points of view on ethical aspects of death and dying, my conclusion is that there is a moral principle to be upheld. Namely, that the deliberate ending of a human life at any stage is objectively wrong. It is on the basis of this principle that nurses and doctors should take clinical decisions regarding their individual patients. Society has yet to reach this ideal in many areas. Is modern warfare ever justifiable? Can judicial execution of a murderer be a good moral choice? A set of negative precepts is unhelpful unless one is prepared to attempt to help in achieving the ideal. For instance, doctors and nurses should not have to carry the strain of uncertain financial provision for adequate palliative care. Scarce resources should not be an argument for euthanasia (Twycross, 1990). In applying moral principles, there will be many grey areas in practice which only those engaged in a particular situation can resolve to the best of their ability.

ACKNOWLEDGEMENTS

I wish to acknowledge the help of Canon Louis Marteau, Director of the Dympna Centre, London, in writing this chapter. Also, Dr J.K. Mason for permission to quote from his book *Human Life and Medical Practice*, and *The Lancet* for permission to quote from Ahronheim and Gasner (1990).

REFERENCES

Ahronheim, J.C. and Gasner, M. (1990) The sloganism of starvation. *Lancet*, **3**(8684), 278–279.

Council of Europe (1976) *Recommendation 779 on the Rights of the Sick and Dying*. 27th Ordinary Session, January.

Council for Europe (1987) Report of the Conference of European Health Ministers. *Ethical and Socio-Cultural Problems Raised by Organ Transplantation.* Paris 16–17th November.

Crump, A. (1990) Fulfilling a living will. *Nursing Standard*, **4**, 46–7.

Dunstan, A.S. and Dunstan, G.R. (eds) (1981) *Dictionary of Medical Ethics*, Darton, Longman and Todd, London.

Gomez, C.F. (1991) *Regulating Death: The Case of the Netherlands*, The Free Press, New York.

Hope, T. (1992) Advance directive about medical treatment. *British Medical Journal*, **30**, 388.

Longley, C. (1993) The feel-good factor is here, and it is not all bad. *Daily Telegraph*, June 4th.

Mason, J.K. (1988) *Human Life and Medical Practice*, Edinburgh University Press, Edinburgh, 30, 48.

Rachels, J. (1975) Active and passive euthanasia. *New England Journal of Medicine*, **292**, 78–80.

Twycross, R.G. (1990) Assisted death: a reply. *Lancet*, **336**, 798.

FURTHER READING

Cassidy, S. (1993) Care of the dying. *Tablet*, **247**, 430–1.

Dawson, J. and Phillips, M. *Ethics and Contemporary Science*, Harvester Press, April 1985.

Drain, G. (Chairman) (1990) Assisted death: Institute of Medical Ethics Working Party on the ethics of prolonging life and assisting death. *Lancet*, **336**, 610–13.

Fletcher, D. (1993) Health Services Correspondent. *Daily Telegraph*, June 30th.

Kaye, P. (1992) *A–Z of Hospice and Palliative Medicine*, EPL Publications, Northampton.

Kelly, K. (1993) Rest for Tony Bland. *Tablet*, **247**, 332–4.

Lamb, D. (1992) *Organ Transplants – Dying, Death and Bereavement*, (eds D. Dickinson and M. Johnson), Sage, London.

Lyall, J. (1991) Final choices. *Nursing Times*, **87**(36), 18–19.

Peter, D. and Sutcliffe, J. (1992) Organ donation: the hospice perspective. *Palliative Medicine*, **6**(3), 212–16.

Pope John Paul II (1993) *Veritatis Splendor* (The Splendour of Truth). Encyclical.

Saunders, C. (1992) Voluntary euthanasia. *Palliative Medicine*, **6**(1), 1–6.

Slack, A. (1992) Killing and allowing to die in medical practice. *Palliative Medicine*, **6**(1).

15 Use of a day centre

This chapter seeks to look at the value of a day centre to the dying patient and their family. Day care for this group of people has grown over the last decade. In a study, 15% of patients being discharged from St Luke's Hospice, Sheffield, following admission for respite or symptom control care were under stress and there was no means at that time of keeping in touch (Wilkes *et al.*, 1978). Patients were also being admitted to the inpatient unit whose spouses would have preferred to continue their care at home and may have been able to do so if there had been the possibility of support from a day centre (Bellamy, 1981). From these beginnings the first day centres in palliative care evolved and there are now many throughout the country.

Centres are called by different names. Some refer to day care, some day centre, others use the term day hospice. Dobratz (1990) states that 'hospice' and 'palliative care' are interchangeable and 'denote the enabling services given to the group of care recipients'. This is the care given to the dying patient and their family and friends. Day care in a hospice is an integral part of that establishment. The philosophy of care is embraced by all. Day hospice is a term used by some units and does, perhaps, bring together the objectives of a hospice day care scheme rather than 'day care' or 'day centre' as provided within the community for other groups of clients.

TYPES OF DAY CENTRE

Independent centre

This is where day care is provided independently from an inpatient unit. It can be in conjunction with a home care service or in cooperation with the Macmillan nursing service. From these centres inpatient units have developed. They fulfil a need for that particular community providing a centre where palliative care services are identified with all that these embrace, such as symptom control advice.

Integrated with inpatient unit

A centre which runs very closely with an inpatient unit. This enables both aspects of the care to supplement and enhance the other. Patients within the hospice meet those attending on a daily basis. This can break down barriers as, in the author's experience, new patients to the day centre may have some fear of a 'hospice' and be wary of accepting an inpatient bed. After attendance on a daily basis and talking to and sharing with the inpatients, many fears are swept away. Inpatients also benefit as on discharge, attendance at the day centre may provide them with a feeling of security, assuring them that contact can be maintained.

Examining the caring behaviour of hospice nurses whilst supporting the patient in the home, as perceived by the caregivers, the fact that the hospice nurses were accessible 24 hours per day reduced the family anxieties (Hull, 1991). Although day care is not a 24-hour service, the fact that it is part of the integrated hospice service does allow for accessibility for advice at any time. This relies on close communication between all staff both formally at the multidisciplinary meeting and on an informal basis.

Satellite centres

In rural areas it has been found to be beneficial to set up satellite centres, such as in Lincolnshire where identified centres are established away from the main centre at St Barnabas' Hospice in Lincoln. This allows for a more effective coverage of a large catchment area (Preston, 1992).

St Clare Trust, run by West Essex Hospice Care, meets in a different place each day of the week. These centres minimize the travelling of the patients who may otherwise be deterred from attending a central location.

STAFFING AND ACCESS

The leadership of day centres varies. Many have nurses but not all. Some are run by physiotherapists, others by occupational therapists. Many rely very heavily on volunteers who provide the centre with a wealth of experience.

Access to centres varies but many use volunteer drivers to transport the patients if their own family are unable to do so. Some centres have their own minibus. The distance and time of the journey can inhibit a few patients if they are not brought directly from their home to the hospice, whilst others will enjoy being out and about. Specialized transport can be an advantage if patients are unable to transfer from a wheelchair to car.

TYPICAL DAY

Centres approach their care from different aspects. Some follow a medical model of care with the medical director attending for consultation whereas others have a more social model. Many are between the two, with the medical director available but not seen on a daily basis.

The day nearly always commences with a renewing of acquaintances and a drink in order to recuperate after the journey. Negotiation may then take place as to the structure of the day ahead. Is the hairdresser or aromatherapist expected that day? Many patients appreciate the individual care – it is not only the women who queue up for the manicurist. Perhaps there is a need to see the doctor or a problem the physiotherapist may be able to solve.

Some centres provide baths for people who cannot manage on their own at home. Some provide the opportunity for dressings to be changed. These cannot be available in centres which are perhaps housed in borrowed facilities such as church halls.

The programmes are varied and may include craft demonstrations, the opportunity to participate in recreational activities such as painting, modelling, needlecraft, woodwork or any other hobbies.

Outings are arranged and vary according to the time of day and the particular wishes of the group of patients but may include coffee mornings, shopping trips, picnic lunches, visits to garden centres or other places of interest. Even a trip to the local supermarket can be enjoyable for somebody who has not been out of the house much lately.

A pub lunch is a popular activity and many people are surprised as to how the most 'normal' of pastimes can bring such pleasure to a group of people who had perhaps felt that their disease prevented them from enjoying these.

Lunchtimes are very social and there is often the offer of an aperitif or perhaps a glass of wine with the meal. For some the fact that the meal is prepared for them, taking into consideration any particular dietary requirements, and that they can enjoy the company of others within an attractively arranged dining room means that they sometimes eat and enjoy it far more than if they were at home.

Relaxation may be taught on a group level or there are tapes available for individuals to use. After lunch there is usually a quiet time and some may even have a sleep! Because the patient is treated independently there are some people who need to rest at other times as well and this may be using a relaxer chair or a bed if there is one available.

Entertainment is arranged and varies from local school children who are pleased to come in to demonstrate their skills to professionals who give their time voluntarily.

The end of the day comes all too quickly for some of the patients. The goodbyes are said over a cup of tea and a piece of cake often shared by relatives and volunteer drivers. This is a valuable time when the staff may get to know the relatives and friends, thus building up a relationship for the future when the loved one dies and support is needed. There is often the need for advice and counselling whilst caring for someone who is getting frailer with some distressing symptoms with which the carer finds it difficult to deal.

Day care does provide respite for carers and enables them to use the time to recharge their batteries in whatever way is applicable to them. Many carers report insufficient sleep. They are up at night with the patient and if they sleep, are anticipating the patient's needs and are not fully relaxed. Many of the carers become isolated within the home with the patient (Decker and Young, 1991). Day care gives the carer time to catch up on sleep or to go out of the house for a few hours. A visit to the dentist, personal shopping that they do not want to ask anybody else to get are all reasons given when considering the advantages of a day care facility.

The author has also found that it provides respite for the patient who may find the intense caring of a loved one smothering and it gives them the opportunity to draw breath and perhaps defuses what could be an explosive situation.

HOLIDAYS

Some centres have ventured into taking patients on holiday, providing an experience that many had thought was beyond their wildest dreams during the terminal stage of an illness. Families enjoy exploration of either old and familiar or new venues whilst supported by the staff from the day care centre. People without close families are helped by volunteers with whom they are familiar from the centre.

Transport can either be in minibuses or private cars but needs careful consideration with regard to different people's limitations. Wheelchairs need to be available so that those who can only mobilize in a limited way can perhaps have their horizons extended.

There is a hotel run by the Macmillan Trust that caters particularly for patients in the terminal stages of cancer. Holidays can be planned at other hotels bearing in mind the special needs of the client group.

NATIONAL ASSOCIATION OF HOSPICE AND PALLIATIVE DAY CARE LEADERS

This was established in 1993 and the aim is to provide a forum for all those involved in day care, thus providing support for leaders who in many cases are working in isolation. Ideas are shared and the annual conference gives delegates the opportunity to meet as well as the educational input.

OTHER CREATIVE ACTIVITIES IN PALLIATIVE CARE

The day centre, in whatever form it takes, is often a resource centre for the arts. Having said that, those concerned with providing care for the dying patient and their family should also look to the local community to see what else is readily available. We need to ensure that all relevant agencies are appropriately involved and that the hospice or palliative care unit makes its own concerns known in the immediate locality.

Within a centre there are often artists, musicians or writers involved, either in a paid or voluntary capacity. Their presence is valuable not least because they approach the concept of care from a different perspective to that of the professional carer and this can add to the dimensions of care provided. If a centre seeks to have a structured commitment to the arts then they may consider sponsorship for an artist in residence or those involved in local authority adult education may be able to assist. However, it is vital that any artist is fully integrated into the team with which they will be working. Those who come in on a weekly or irregular basis can often feel rather isolated from the daily round and there should be a firm support system *in situ*.

Whatever the 'professional' input the talents and skills of the staff, patients, volunteers and relatives should be drawn on as much as possible for within the existing framework there is always a rich seam of inspiration and talent. As patients do not belong to some homogeneous group with common interests, the better the understanding of the various cultures and communities from which they come, the more appropriate will be the activities that take place within a centre. There is a need for flexibility, enthusiasm and good communication between all those involved. In an ideal situation those concerned with the arts will be able to take their expertise onto the wards and indeed into people's homes to encourage and help with particular interests when people are unable or unwilling to visit a centre.

The reasons for a person becoming involved are personal and varied. Some may simply want to continue an interest that has been part of their previous lifestyle. Others may wish to leave a 'mark' that will remain after they have died – poems, paintings and pottery have all been undertaken for this purpose (although this is seldom stated specifically). One person made up and recorded stories for his children to listen to when he would no longer be there to talk to them himself. Others have written poems when deep feelings and emotions are hard to express in general conversation: 'Imagery and symbolism come to the rescue when it is too difficult to speak of profound or frightening things and, positively, they may lead to new thoughts or layers of meaning' (Gloag, 1990). Reminiscence, the desire to tell one's own story, is also a motivating factor: 'Sometimes a piece of writing would result, sometimes the telling was enough' (Hawes, 1991).

The very act of creating can give back to a person a sense of achievement and self-esteem when so much is being lost: 'Having a sense of purpose and a feeling of self-worth is in itself therapeutic, leading us to venture further in developing our own potential' (Frampton, 1986). By encouraging people to try something new the distress felt at the decline of a previously held skill can sometimes be alleviated – someone who is no longer able to knit, perhaps because of weakness in one hand, may be interested in learning to weave.

Although the benefits of creative activities such as writing, painting, piano playing (keyboards with headphones are a boon on wards) are considerable, one has to guard against the idea that 'a busy patient is a happy patient'. The more passive dimensions of the arts are often more appropriate when working with people who are very ill, sometimes bored but often weary. It is important to ensure that the painting or photographs on the wall, facing the bed or the chair, give pleasure to the person who is looking at them. Individual tastes in music can easily be catered for by encouraging people to consider listening to tapes but when it is possible to have live music, which gives much pleasure, care needs to be taken that the personal preference of the provider does not obscure the interests of those in receipt of the provision.

There are local and national organizations who have experience in performing in hospitals and hospices. Both drama and music are available through these agencies (see Useful Addresses). Schools and colleges in the area are often delighted to come and entertain and this can be an ideal way for the local community to become involved with a centre. However, it is important that those visiting from outside are fully aware of the nature of the care provided and the vulnerability of some of the audience. Ideally an initial visit will take place prior to the performance and at very least the proposed programme will be discussed. The performers also need a 'debriefing' session after the event so that they can discuss their own feelings about the visit.

Some hospices and palliative care units employ art, music or drama therapists. These are trained professionals: 'At present, criteria for involving the music therapist include extreme anxiety, alarming withdrawal, language barriers, difficulties of interaction and intractable pain . . .' (Munro and Mount, 1978). The reasons for involvement are not always so severe and there are certainly times when a therapist is appropriate. But we need to beware of inappropriate use of the term 'therapy'. Often it is tagged on to any activity undertaken by those who are seriously ill or disabled. This not only detracts from the work of the qualified therapist but serves to reinforce the 'patientness' of the person in receipt of care. To say that someone who is simply painting for pleasure is doing 'art therapy' suggests they are no longer able, or expected, to take delight in usual activities.

One of the most relevant and essential aspects of the arts in palliative care is a comprehensive library service. If possible, use the local library services and see if the housebound or mobile service will include the centre in its provision. This means that there will be access to books in several languages, books that are only available in other libraries, large print books and some books on tape. Many libraries offer videos, paintings, music tapes and information about other services in the local vicinity. They will also be able to visit people in their own homes.

When asked if they enjoy reading, many people reply that they used to but they don't seem to be able to concentrate any more. This lack of concentration is often due to sheer weariness. If they agree to try large print books they are often able to enjoy reading again. There is sometimes a stigma attached to requesting large print and the offer of it as first choice makes a tremendous difference. It is also useful to have access to, and information on, books on tape (see Useful Addresses) as, although the libraries can provide them, the selection is sometimes limited.

The arts, whether considered from a creative, diversional or environmental perspective, should be an integral part of palliative care and not some cosmetic appendage. Each unit or centre will have its own agenda which will reflect and integrate the interests of those being cared for and the particular skills of the carers. Where there are young children in a family, including them in activities can help them feel more involved and those who are bereaved may be able to express their grief through writing or painting. Ideally a 'menu' of ideas and suggestions is offered to the patient and their family so that they are aware of what is possible, if they are interested. However, it is crucially important that all those concerned should feel comfortable if they choose to do nothing at all.

REFERENCES

Bellamy, S. (1981) A day care system to support the terminally ill, in *Cancer Nursing Update. Proceedings of the 2nd International Cancer Nursing Conference* (ed. R. Tiffany), Baillière Tindall, London, pp. 62–4.

Decker, S.D. and Young, E. (1991) Self-perceived needs of primary care givers of home–hospice clients. *Journal of Community Health Nursing*, **8**(3), 147–54.
Dobratz, M.C. (1990) Hospice nursing. Present perspectives and future directives. *Cancer Nursing*, **13**(2), 116–22.
Frampton, D. (1986) Restoring creativity to the dying patient. *British Medical Journal*, **293**, 1593.
Gloag, D. (1990) Death is no longer a stranger. *British Medical Journal*, **300**, 1214.
Hawes, C. (1991) Writing in residence. *British Medical Journal*, **303**, 527.
Hull, M.M. (1991) Hospice nurses. Caring support for caregiving families. *Cancer Nursing*, **14**(2), 63–70.
Munro, S. and Mount, B. (1978) Music therapy in palliative care. *CMA Journal*, **119**, 259.
Preston, K. (1992) Satellite programme. Day care expansion in Lincolnshire. *Day Care Newsletter*, October 1992.
Wilkes, E., Crowther, A.G.O. and Greaves. C.W.K.H. (1978) A different kind of day hospital – for patients with preterminal cancer and chronic disease. *British Medical Journal*, **2**, 1053–6.

FURTHER READING

Corr, C.A. and Corr, D.M. (1991) Adult hospice day care. *Death Studies*, **16**(2), 155–71.

USEFUL ADDRESSES

The Actors' Centre, 4 Chenies Street, London WC1 7EP
Tel. 071 631 3619

British Health Care, Arts Centre, The College of Art, Perth Road, Dundee DD1 4HT
Tel. 0382 23261

Calibre (Talking Books for The Blind), New Road, Weston Turville, Aylesbury HP22 5XQ
Tel. 0296 432339

Council for Music in Hospitals, 74 Queens Road, Surrey KT12 5LW
Tel. 0932 252809

National Listening Library, 12 Lant Street, London SE1 1QH
Tel. 071 407 9417

RNIB Talking Book Service, Mount Pleasant, Wembley HA0 1RR
Tel. 081 903 6666

16 Care in the home

Many patients with a terminal illness express a desire to die at home (Townsend *et al.*, 1990). Here they can remain within the security of a known environment, surrounded by family and friends and be cared for by the family general practitioner. At home there is more opportunity for the patient to have greater control over decision making and life is not being dictated by the endless routines found in busy hospital wards. Household noises are familiar and less likely to disturb sleep, unlike those made by the clanking of bedpans, drug rounds or the confused patient in the bed next door. Families are not restricted to visiting hours and the patient's diet will often be more accommodating to their particular needs and fancies on each day. Familiarity is comforting and contributes towards a feeling of safety and belonging. However, perhaps most importantly, dying at home enables the individual to continue to be seen as a person and not just as another patient in another hospital bed.

Baddeley (1991) suggests that 'the time of death is not usually within our control, the manner of dying may be, but the place of death often is'. However, it remains that death continues to occur frequently within institutions (Field and James, 1993; Townsend *et al.*, 1990). The reasons for this may be varied. Patients who have been through vigorous treatments requiring extended periods of time spent on a particular ward may prefer to return to an environment where they are known to the staff and have trust and confidence in them. Some patients and carers feel more secure in the knowledge that there are medical and nursing staff in attendance 24 hours a day, which is seldom found in the community setting. Carers may be absent or may not have sufficient emotional, physical or domestic resources to permit them to look after the individual into the terminal stages of the illness. A poor understanding or denial of the situation often makes it difficult for plans to be made towards the inevitability of reduced independence and loss of function. Poor communication with the primary care team as a result of stress, anger, denial and fear will inhibit open discussion, exploration of problems and examination of options available to improve quality of life and care at home. As a result symptoms remain uncontrolled, carers become worn out, tempers become frayed and fears remain unexplored and unchallenged. Consequently admission is often the response to change and crisis.

It must not be forgotten that caring for the dying patient at home and supporting relatives can be very stressful to the professional carer. Many doctors and nurses continue to feel inadequately prepared for this role. Admission to hospital may prove an easier option to the discomfort and frustration of not feeling able to meet the ever-changing needs of the dying patient and the family. Education remains paramount to successful care at home. Lorraine Sherr (1989) suggests that 'training should therefore address both the stresses that are associated with the provision of care as well as an understanding of how best to provide care in situations of loss'.

THE IMPACT OF ILLNESS UPON THE PATIENT AND FAMILY

Serious illness brings about a great many changes in the lives of both patient and family. In the early stages of ill health it may be that these changes are slight, with little impact on daily activities. To outward appearances the patient may appear reasonably well. However, from the point of realization of failing health and diagnosis, the person's life has become irrevocably changed. The patient and family are now living with the uncertainty of future events and the threat of separation. There is often a feeling of chaos and a sense of loss of control.

As the disease progresses and the patient's condition begins to deteriorate there is an ever-increasing experience of loss. The patient may express feelings of low self-esteem, worthlessness and helplessness. There may be feelings of no longer having their established place within the family or society. Jobs may have been given up, careers and ambitions curtailed and roles within the family changed. Children, in particular the young, may be excluded from receiving information in an attempt to protect them from pain and distress. Alternatively, greater responsibility and expected maturity may have befallen the older children with the family. Expectations upon them may be high, in addition to pressures that might already be present in the form of school examinations or new jobs. Although illness primarily affects the individual with the disease, its effects reach out and touch the lives of all those people close to and sometimes distant from the patient.

A sense of isolation is very common to people facing the prospect of death. This can be increased as contact with the hospital becomes less frequent, when a general practitioner or district nurse fail to visit the home or friends call less often. But perhaps the greatest feeling of isolation can occur as a result of a conspiracy of silence within the family itself. This is often due to a desire by family members to protect each other and themselves from painful but honest conversations about the illness and the future. It is unfortunate that this should occur at a time when sharing, touching and support is vital to so many in order to reduce the overwhelming burden of living with terminal illness.

With this in mind, what can the nurse offer the patient and family? We can offer them *interest*, *time*, *honesty*, *reliability* and *availability*. It is important to demonstrate that as professionals we care about what is happening to them. That they are not simply being labelled as people for whom no more can be done. That we are prepared to give time to listen to their feelings, fears and anxieties and that we will approach them with openness and honesty. This can be done without forcing information upon them that they are not ready to receive. It is essential that the nurse is reliable in the service that they are offering to the patient. Too often patients who have been through palliative treatments or those for whom no treatment has been available express feelings of being let down by health care professionals. We must also ensure that we are available to them, not just at the time of our visit to their home but also at other times should a problem arise. This can be particularly important at night when fears may be heightened and symptoms exacerbated. At this time it is usually the general practitioner or locum doctor who is on call; however, in some areas there may also be twilight or night nursing services. Sometimes the availability of someone to talk to on the phone and the knowledge that someone cares may be sufficient to reduce anxiety until a visit is made the following day.

ASSESSMENT

Assessment assists us in identifying the needs of the patient and family and enables us to set goals and plan care. It is a continuous process throughout contact with the patient and needs regular review and evaluation.

The initial assessment is one of the most important visits made to the patient. It is then that the foundation stone for our relationship is established. It must never be hurried and work should be planned in order to allow sufficient time to listen, exchange information and outline a plan of care. If possible the patient should be contacted prior to the visit in order to give them time to prepare themselves and to invite another family member to be present if desired. The nurse should ensure that they have as much information as possible prior to making the visit by liaising with the relevant professionals such as the general practitioner, the hospital or hospital support teams.

Assessment begins before meeting the patient. Taking note of the local environment can often give an indication of potential difficulties the patient might experience during their illness. Is the area well served by local shops that the carer can get to easily without having to leave the patient for extended periods of time? Is it a house or a tower block, in which case what sort of access is there? Are there stairs, lifts, ramps for wheelchair use? In some areas parking facilities can be very poor and this may be important when considering the delivery of equipment at a later date.

Once inside the home information can be obtained in several ways: by conversation, observation and the use of our senses. The extent of the assessment will be determined by the circumstances the nurse finds on arrival. For example, if the patient is in great pain or extremely anxious, the nurse may have to tailor their questioning to the most important facts or rely heavily upon the family to give details. A full assessment does not necessarily have to take place at this first visit. It may take time before the patient gains sufficient trust to feel comfortable in talking about feelings or more intimate aspects of their lives and their care.

By listening to the patient's account of the events leading up to and beyond diagnosis it is possible to get a basic knowledge of the person's present medical history and treatment. It also gives us an idea of what the patient and family have been going through and often serves to give some indication of their insight into the disease. It can be very interesting to note the terminology used by the patient when describing their illness as this may reveal the degree of acceptance or understanding about the disease. Terms such as shadow on the lung, a black ulcer, growth, tumour or cancer may be used.

Once rapport has been established the nurse can begin to explore how the illness is affecting them now. What do the patient and carer identify as the problems at present and how do they see themselves being helped? This will include problems associated with unpleasant symptoms of the disease and possibly its treatments and also how the illness is affecting their day-to-day lives. It may be that by the end of the visit there are many different, apparently urgent problems or concerns. It may not be possible or wise to attempt to deal with them all at once. In this case it is important that the patient is able to discuss and identify which should take priority and realistic goals set.

Other useful information will include relevant past medical history and a list of current medication and any known allergies. With this the nurse will be able to assess the effectiveness of present drug therapies and to note any side effects. Commonly patients who are dying find themselves taking endless amounts of tablets, some of which may no longer be beneficial. The nurse may find themselves acting as the patient's advocate in identifying when there is difficulty in taking medication. By discussion with the general practitioner it may be that some of these medications can be omitted or more convenient routes of administration found, i.e. sub-lingual, rectal or via a syringe driver.

In hospital it is often difficult for patients to refuse medication as they may be fearful of offending the doctor or causing trouble. At home the individual has a lot more control and can take the decision to stop medications if desired. Common reasons for poor compliance at home are too many tablets, fear and misunderstanding about the purpose of the drugs or simply that the patient feels too weak or uncomfortable to be bothered. Introducing a drug chart which explains the reasons for use and indicates how and when to take the medication can do much to relieve anxiety and reduce confusion. It can also be very helpful when the patient is attending outpatient appointments or when requesting repeat prescriptions from the general practitioner. All medications are the property of the patient for whom they have been prescribed. However the nurse has a responsibility to ensure that the patient and carer are aware of how to administer the drugs correctly and how to store them safely (UKCC, 1992).

As discussed earlier it is important to recognize the person within the patient. This further enables us to understand how the illness might be affecting them and helps us to begin to appreciate the losses they are encountering. Getting to know the patient and family and gaining their trust will take time. This will not be achieved in a single visit. It may be helpful to know what line of work someone used to do and how they felt about it, how they may have coped with retirement, redundancy or having to give up their job as a result of their ill health. Noting their likes, dislikes, hobbies and ambitions will help to demonstrate to them our interest and concern for them as individuals and increase our understanding of their needs.

Establishing who are the family and friends most important to the patient and where they live helps us to begin to create the picture of the person's life. Drawing a family tree permits us to see at a glance who is around the patient and most likely to be affected by the illness. Being aware of the ages of the family members, their occupations, health needs and family relationships increases the likelihood of us meeting the needs of both the patient and carers.

CARE OF THE PATIENT

Much has been written about the nursing care of the dying patient in previous chapters of this book. The principles remain the same for patients dying at home, but the approach may need to be slightly more imaginative and flexible. The nurse may well encounter insufficient resources, delays in obtaining specialized equipment and home environments that are not always conducive to providing quality care. As a person becomes weaker tasks such as walking around the home, negotiating stairs or getting washed and dressed in the mornings can become increasingly daunting. With the help of the district nurse and the community occupational therapist these tasks can be made easier and safer. This can be achieved by the introduction of aids and adaptions such as a handrail on the stairs or by the bath or toilet. A walking stick or a Zimmer frame may help to support and give confidence to someone who is frail and weak. A wheelchair may enable the individual to be taken out and help to alleviate some of the boredom that can occur from spending continuous time at home. A low chair, bed or toilet can be very difficult to get up from if a person lacks energy or feels uncomfortable. Simple adaptions such as bed blocks, chair and toilet raisers can often enable the patient to negotiate these with more ease and comfort.

As the patient's condition deteriorates it is obvious that longer lengths of time are spent in bed. This can become very isolating if the bedroom is upstairs away from everyday activities. It may be more convenient for both the patient and the carer to have the bed brought downstairs, perhaps into the living room. This enables the individual to remain part of the family life and to be aware of and involved in things happening around them. However, it can also mean less privacy and reveals to family and friends that the person is unwell and losing independence. This may not be acceptable to some patients who prefer to maintain the impression that nothing is amiss. For this reason great sensitivity is required when suggesting changes around the home or introducing equipment such as commodes and bedtables. The patient may not yet be ready to accept being less able to undertake daily routine activities and certainly may not want this made common knowledge to anyone who might come to the house. It must be remembered that this is the patient's home and the nurse is the guest. It is not a hospital ward to be cluttered up with equipment that might never be used.

With increasing weakness comes greater dependency upon others for care and support. Families will need advice, supervision and encouragement at this time. Carers are often frightened at the prospect of having to maintain the patient's need for personal hygiene. If acceptable, the nurse can demonstrate how to maintain privacy and warmth and to make an assessment of need based on the patient's wishes and general condition. Patients who are uncomfortable or dying seldom want to be disturbed and usually a basic wash is all that is required to keep a person fresh and maintain their dignity. For some patients and carers the intimacy of such care may be unacceptable. For others this task may prove to be too difficult for either emotional or physical reasons. In these cases the district nurse can arrange for a nurse or care attendant to attend to these basic needs.

Weakness and reduced mobility increase the risk of developing pressure sores. A variety of pressure relieving apparatus is usually available within the local health authority such as Spenco or large cell ripple mattresses, sheepskins or Spenco cushions. These can usually be obtained via the district nurse or occupational therapist. Advising the patient and family on the importance of skin care and pressure relief is essential if the patient is to remain comfortable at home and minimize the risk of developing soreness.

Patients with advanced malignant disease often experience taste and appetite changes and diet commonly becomes the focus of attention (Twycross and Lack, 1990). There may be a tendency for the carer to try and 'build up' the individual by encouraging food throughout the day. Strong cooking smells, fatty foods and too much on a plate may be very off-putting to someone who is feeling nauseous or has no appetite. Suggesting small portions, attractively presented and appetizing to the patient may be of some benefit. A variety of food supplement drinks, many of which are available on prescription, can be taken in place of or in addition to meals but should never be forced upon the individual.

Cooking for someone at home can be seen as a way of doing something constructive to help the patient but too often it simply becomes a source of tension. Patients may feel pressurized and guilty at not eating what has been carefully and lovingly prepared. Carers become increasingly frustrated, angry and frightened at the repeated throwing away of meals and being unable to prevent further weight loss and deterioration. Once again the nurse may have to act as the patient's advocate in assisting the carer to understand that due to advancing disease and increasing inactivity, the person is no longer able to manage the meals as they once used to. It may be appropriate to try and divert attention towards something more beneficial to the patient at this time, such as sips of fluid or mouth care. This will help the carer to feel they still have a positive part to play and reintroduces an element of control at a time of great change.

BALANCE OF CARE

In order for our support to be successful it is important that we aim for a balance of care. Maslow (1943) identified a hierarchy of needs starting with those necessary for survival and finishing with those connected with self-actualization. These include physiological needs, safety needs, belongingness and love needs, esteem needs and the need for self-actualization.

When caring for the dying patient it is important that all these needs are considered and attempts made to assist the patient to meet them. It would be of limited value if we concerned ourselves solely with symptomatic relief if what the patient was really worrying about was how their family were going to cope or more simply how they were going to be able to walk the dog as they become less well. There needs to be a balance of symptom control, psychological support and practical care and advice. This holistic approach centres around the patient and upon their priority of needs. That is not to say that what we perceive to be a problem should be disregarded. On the contrary, it should be discussed with the patient and if desired, incorporated into the planning of care alongside the patient's priorities.

The patient's condition may rapidly change with progression of the disease. Hence the plan of care needs to be adaptable and reviewed on a regular basis. Anticipating needs rather than dealing later with a problem is the key to successful care planning. Where possible all care should be discussed with the patient and family. Information and explanations should be offered to increase understanding and help to empower the patient at a time of their feeling most helpless. Much has been written about the use of nursing models as guidelines for the planning and delivery of care in a variety of nursing contexts. It may be necessary for the nurse to examine the strengths and weaknesses of the particular model being used in the area in order to ensure that it is the most appropriate way of providing effective care for the dying patient and their family at home.

It would be wrong to look solely at the needs of the patient in isolation from the family, who are often in attendance for long periods of time. This is not only physically but emotionally draining and difficult to sustain in isolation. In the past it was more common for families to be familiar with illness and death at home. Today, however, carers often have little experience in looking after someone who is seriously ill and may feel insecure about their role as caregiver. Consequently the nurse has a large part to play in teaching, advising and encouraging the carer in this new and often frightening role. If care at home is to be maintained it is important that the nurse utilizes resources within the family and assists them in developing positive coping strategies (Bond, 1986). Each family is unique and will respond to the challenge in differing ways, some requiring more assistance and time than others.

Not everyone has a carer or family who feel able to take on this role. This can be for many reasons, for example, ill health, other family commitments, travelling distance, fear and insecurity or simply that it is not felt to be their responsibility. It is important to listen to what the family/carers are saying, to explore any fears and identify options open to them. If the patient lives alone or family feel unable to participate in the care, then even greater emphasis must be placed upon the primary care team and social services available in the area.

CARE OF THE FAMILY

Caring for a relative who is dying at home can place tremendous strain upon a family. Lives are disrupted and usual routines abandoned. Relatives may have to give up work in order to be in constant attendance on the patient. For some this may be a natural and desired course of events but for others the restriction upon their lives and social activities may be inconvenient and unwanted. Many relatives are keen to support the person who is dying and this is often a way of expressing their care and concern. However, some people find themselves in the role of caregiver out of necessity or a sense of duty. Feelings may be very mixed and confused. Relatives may feel frightened, overburdened and resentful at being forced into a situation over which there seems no control.

Friction may develop between family members. This may be through a sense of rivalry over who should act as the main carer or as a result of too much responsibility being placed upon one individual. Families under stress often fail to recognize their united strength and consequently their care and time giving may be haphazard and unsupportive to the patient. A family meeting with a member of the primary care team may prove a useful way of approaching problems, exploring fears and encouraging the family to examine ways in which their time and support may be more effectively distributed. It is important, however, to appreciate that some families will interact harmoniously but in others there will be rifts and antagonism which may be of many years duration. Life-threatening illness within a family can sometimes act as a catalyst to building bridges and enhancing relationships that have previously been poor. Alternatively anxiety and high levels of emotion can result in further disharmony and alienation. In this instance it would be futile to expect a family to work together for any length of time. Members will need to be supported individually or alternative arrangements made for the care of the patient at home.

Attention and concern tend to focus upon the person who is dying and too often the needs of the carer are not adequately recognized. It is important to acknowledge their contribution to the care and the difficulties they are having to deal with on a daily basis. Carers greatly appreciate being asked how they are and how they feel they are managing. They need time to share their feelings and explore their fears. Difficulties can arise when a patient and family have been given an expected prognosis. When this occurs there is a tendency for families to put all their energy reserves into this period and adjust their lives accordingly. If the patient then outlives this prognosis families may well feel confused and angry at being 'misled' by professionals. Feelings of guilt are common as they wonder how much longer the patient will live and they may find themselves wishing it was all over. Alternatively the patient and family may feel cheated and angry when deterioration occurs before the predicted time.

Previous experience of trauma and loss will often affect one's ability to cope with the present situation (Parkes, 1978). If a relative's experience of death is one of pain and suffering it will be natural to anticipate this as the course of events to come. It is important to allow time to explore past experiences and to offer reassurance of close monitoring and control of symptoms and availability of professional help at all times. Many carers are apprehensive about what to expect as death approaches and will commonly be guided and sometimes misled by friends and neighbours. Relatives need to be kept informed of the patient's condition and given information about what to expect, in order to prepare themselves for the future events. Much anxiety can be relieved by explaining changes in levels of consciousness and breathing prior to death. During this time carers may feel uncertain about what to do. Where possible they should be encouraged to continue to talk to and sit with the patient and undertake simple tasks such as mouth care and pressure area relief.

It is common for relatives to feel that they have to keep strong. It is important for us to give them permission to cry and to express their feelings. Acknowledging emotions is essential to relieve the tension and the pressure that may be present. Too often the care of the patient is at the expense of the carer. On enquiry one may find that the carer is not eating or sleeping properly and is not having any time to themselves. If there are other family members or friends it may be possible for them to arrange to stay with the patient for a few hours during the day. This will allow the carer to go out shopping, to visit friends or simply to have the time to be alone. Alternatively help can be sought from the Marie Curie Nursing Service. This organization can provide a nurse trained in cancer care to stay with a patient for up to 24 hours in order to give the carer a break or a chance to sleep.

From April 1993 the National Health Service and Community Care Act requires social service departments to make assessment for the provision of individualized packages of care for patients in the community. Availability to help will vary from area to area. There may be home care assistants or aides who will be available to sit with a patient for short periods of time. The use of Meals on Wheels, home help and laundry services may be of benefit to some patients. Some areas will have voluntary organizations such as Crossroads Care Attendant Schemes who have home care attendants trained in basic nursing and whose aim is to support carers at home. For some individuals this type of help may be sufficient to allow them to relax and recuperate. For others longer periods of time away from the caring role may be required. This can be met either in the form of day centre facilities or respite admissions.

Many hospices, hospitals and nursing homes have facilities for short term stay of one or two weeks in order to give carers a break or sometimes to address symptoms that are proving difficult to control at home. For many patients and families the availability of respite care in one form or another will make the difference between coping or not coping at home.

Reduced finances and extra expenses will increase the strain upon the family and patient. If desired, they can be referred to a social worker or Citizens Advice Bureau for information and advice on entitlement to social security benefits. Grants may be available for people with cancer and other illnesses from organizations such as Cancer Relief Macmillan Fund and Counsel and Care for the Elderly.

MULTIDISCIPLINARY APPROACH AND COMMUNICATION

Caring for someone who is dying at home requires a multidisciplinary approach. This incorporates the skills of differing professionals, statutory and voluntary organizations. The nurse should be aware of and understand the roles, functions and responsibilities of other team members, other professionals and other agencies. They should know when it is appropriate to seek advice and how to make a referral.

The general practitioner and district nurse usually have a key role in the care of the terminally ill at home. However, they are often supported by other professionals such as social workers, occupational therapists, physiotherapists and specialist nurses or teams. Many hospitals now have palliative care support teams who will get to know patients and families at some point during hospital admissions. They offer support and symptom control and can provide a useful link between hospital and community. In most areas there are now a number of specialist nurses working alongside the community staff in order to meet the needs of people living at home with a variety of medical conditions. Their advice or supervision can be invaluable in improving quality of life for the patient and family within the community setting. Macmillan nurses are specially trained in pain and symptom control. Their role is that of advice, information and support to patients with cancer and their carers, as well as to their professional colleagues. Many of these nurses are now working within multidisciplinary teams. Their support is intended to complement that provided by the primary care team and hospitals and should not displace any of these caring professions.

Good communication is essential in order to ensure that care is effective and to minimize the risk of confusion between professional colleagues. Information exchange must be accurate and occur at regular intervals. This will help to ensure that all parties are aware of changes in the patient's condition, their present needs and the treatments currently being given. In the community setting this is not always easy, particularly if the professionals are not based at the same locality. Much of the liaison takes place via the telephone as this is an easy and quick method of communication. However, all calls should be documented if information is to be retained and of use at a later date. Written communication is also an effective means of keeping up to date although confidentiality must be respected at all times. Letters should be kept safely in patient records and access permitted only to individuals entitled to see them. Face to face contact or case conferences are a particularly useful way of pooling knowledge, assessing needs and making collective plans for care. When more than one agency is involved it is important that there are common goals and that conflicting advice is not being given to the patient and family.

The approach to documenting information varies from area to area but it is common to find patient records in the home as well as within the nursing office. Information kept at home is obviously accessible to the patient and family. Whenever possible all reports should be discussed openly with the patient in order to prevent misunderstanding, misinterpretation and to promote participation in the planning and delivery of care.

WHAT TO DO AFTER SOMEONE DIES

There is usually some indication that death is approaching and this further enables us to prepare the family for this event. It is difficult to predict exact times and it may be important to suggest calling other members of the family, sooner rather than later, if they wish to be in attendance at this time. For some families the support of the local clergy may be of great comfort in assisting them through this stressful period. Respect and sensitivity towards a person's religious or cultural beliefs is essential throughout the illness. It may be necessary to enquire as to whether there are specific needs or requirements that should be met prior to and after the death in order to prevent misunderstanding or interfering with cultural traditions.

Many relatives are frightened by not knowing how they might react once the person has died. There is often a fear that they might panic or 'go to pieces'. Families should be reassured that at this time all they need to do is to contact the general practitioner or attending doctor. Recommending keeping the telephone number clearly visible by the phone will prevent some of the panic about whom to call and may reduce the temptation to dial 999 for an ambulance. Once a person has died it is necessary for the doctor to certify the death and make plans for issuing a medical certificate stating the cause of death. If the individual is to be cremated then the signatures of two doctors are required. If the death was seen to be very unexpected or caused by an industrial disease a post-mortem examination may be needed.

It is not always necessary to perform full Last Offices at home as this is done later by the undertakers. However, the body should be laid flat, the eyes closed, dentures replaced (if desired by the family) and a pillow positioned beneath the chin in order to close the mouth. A full bladder can be emptied by gently pressing above the pubic bone. Catheters, syringe drivers, etc. should be removed at this time. As a last act of care and respect it may be appropriate to wash the body and provide clean clothing. Some families may wish to participate in this or do it by themselves.

Following the death relatives are usually shocked and feel numbed. Each individual will react differently. Some will cry, some will express anger or denial and others may simply withdraw and become silent. Expressions of grief should always be encouraged and the use of sedatives avoided unless absolutely necessary. All relatives and children should have the opportunity to see and say goodbye to the individual should they wish to do so. At this time they may feel supported by the nurse accompanying them back into the room where the death has taken place. Alternatively the family may wish to be alone in order to express their grief in private.

Once the doctor has certified the death, the undertakers can be contacted and arrangements made for the removal of the body to the mortuary. Some families will have selected a funeral director prior to the death but others may need guidance and assistance at this time. Addresses can be found in the Yellow Pages of the telephone directory.

The next days are generally very busy for the family dealing with practicalities. The death should be registered by the Registrar of Births and Deaths for the area in which it occurred. Following this the family will be issued with a certificate for burial or cremation, a certificate of registration of death for social security purposes and a death certificate which is a certified copy of the entry in the death register. The latter will be necessary for applying for funeral grants, pension and insurance claims, etc. at a later date.

Families often request that equipment used during the care is removed from the home as soon as possible and preferably prior to the funeral. Great distress can be caused for the bereaved person who continues to look at a commode several weeks after the death has occurred.

Assessment of bereavement needs is a continuous process. It begins at the initial point of contact with the patient and family and extends into the period after the death. It has been suggested that until the practical issues following a death have been dealt with, the bereaved person may not have the emotional energy to confront difficult feelings and reactions following the loss (Pardoe, 1991). Further information about bereavement can be found in Chapter 20.

REFERENCES

Baddeley, P.G. (1991) A place to die: home, hospice or hospital? *Geriatric Medicine*, **21**(5), 14.
Bond, M. (1986) *Stress and Self-Awareness: A Guide for Nurses*, Butterworth Heinemann, London, pp. 10–13.
Field, D. and James, N. (1993) Where and how people die, in *The Future for Palliative Care*, (ed. D. Clark), Open University Press, Buckingham, pp. 6–29.
Maslow, A.H. (1943) A theory of human motivation. *Psychological Review*, **50**, 370–96.
Pardoe, J. (1991) *How Many Times Can You Say Goodbye?* Triangle/SPCK, London, p. 93.
Parkes, C.M. (1978) *Bereavement – Studies of Grief in Adult Life*, Penguin, Harmondsworth.
Sherr, L. (ed.) (1989) *Death, Dying and Bereavement*, Blackwell Scientific Publications, Oxford, p. 48.
Townsend, J., Frank, A.O., Fermont, D. *et al.* (1990) Terminal cancer care and patients' preference for place of death: a prospective study. *British Medical Journal*, **301**, 415–17.
Twycross, R.G. and Lack, S.A. (1990) *Therapeutics in Terminal Cancer*, 2nd edn, Churchill Livingstone, Edinburgh, p. 47.
United Kingdom Central Council for Nursing, Health Visiting and Midwifery (1992) *Standards for the Administration of Medicines*, UKCC, London.

FURTHER READING

Aggleton, P. and Chalmers, H. (1990) *Nursing Models and the Nursing Process*, Macmillan Education, Basingstoke.
Burns, N., Carney, K. and Brobst, B. (1989) Hospice: a design for home care for the terminally ill. *Holistic Nursing Practice*, **3**(2), 65–76.
Copperman, H. (1983) *Dying at Home*, John Wiley and Sons, Chichester.
Department of Social Security (1990) *What to Do After a Death*, Leaflet D49, HMSO, London.
Dobson, S.M. (1991) *Transcultural Nursing*, Scutari Press, London.
Doyle, D. (1987) *Domiciliary Terminal Care*, Churchill Livingstone, Edinburgh.
Dunlop, R.J. and Hockley, J.M. (1990) *Terminal Care Support Teams*, Oxford University Press, New York.
Dunlop, R.J., Davies, R.J. and Hockley, J.M. (1989) Preferred versus actual place of death: a hospital palliative care support team experience. *Palliative Medicine*, **3**, 197–201.
Dunphy, K.P. and Amesbury, B.D.W. (1990) A comparison of hospice and home care patients: patterns of referral, patient characteristics and predictors of place of death. *Palliative Medicine*, **4**, 105–11.
Hector, W. and Whitfield, S. (1982) *Nursing Care for the Dying Patient and Family*, Heinemann Medical, London.
Jay, P. (1990) Relatives caring for the terminally ill. *Nursing Standard*, **5**, 30–2.

Jones, R. (1992) Primary health care: what should we do for people dying at home with cancer? *European Journal of Cancer Care*, **1**(4), 9–11.

Logan, M. (1988) Care of the terminally ill, includes the family (using the Ray model). *Infirmiere Canadienne*, **84**(5), 30–2, 34.

Mudditt, H. (1987) Home truths (families looking after a terminally ill patient at home need help and advice). *Nursing Times and Nursing Mirror*, **83**, 31–3.

National Health Service and Community Care Act (1990), HMSO, London.

Richardson, J. (1993) *A Death in the Family*, Lion Publishing, Oxford.

Saunders, C. and Sykes, N. (1993) *The Management of Terminal Malignant Disease*, Edward Arnold, London.

Thorpe, G. (1993) Enabling more dying people to remain at home. *British Medical Journal*, **307**, 915–18.

Woodhall, C. (1986) A family concern (is it better to die at home or in hospital?). *Nursing Times and Nursing Mirror*, **82**, 31–3.

Nursing care of the dying patient in hospital

17

Despite the emergence of hospices all over the country it is a well-known fact that a higher percentage of cancer patients die in hospital rather than in hospices or at home (OPCS, 1980).

Why is this so? Admission to hospice is a 'planned admission' but admission to hospital can be obtained as an emergency. The relative has only to dial 999 and the patient can be whisked away to the nearest hospital; they may have to wait their turn in the casualty department but they are in an institution where they feel secure. They may be well known to the physician or surgeon who may have said to them in the outpatient clinic 'You may return at any time' and this is sometimes said without making reference to any interim palliative care at home.

It is a denial of advancing disease that usually provokes an emergency admission from home where the patient and their family are unable to cope any longer due to the lack of availability of community and GP services. To the uninformed great fear is engendered by the mention of hospice care; to some it is so final, it seems like a one-way ticket from which there is no return.

Ignorance of the philosophy of the modern hospice movement means that time, tact and reassurance are needed to explain it to elderly patients. Little do they realize that their care, and that of their relatives, would be greatly enhanced.

Hospital beds are a precious and expensive commodity but that is not necessarily a good reason for transferring a patient to hospice against their will or that of their family.

Patients are therefore admitted to hospital for terminal care because they and their relatives are no longer able to cope physically or emotionally. There is usually a crisis at home with exacerbation of symptoms or a trauma necessitating emergency admission. Dunlop and Hockley (1990) found that patients admitted to hospital had a variety of untreated symptoms:

1. pain
2. anorexia
3. constipation
4. insomnia
5. weakness and malaise
6. dyspnoea
7. nausea and vomiting
8. cough
9. oedema
10. sore mouth
11. agitation and confusion
12. dysphagia.

So often these symptoms are poorly managed '. . . because the patients do not complain, professionals fail to appreciate the symptoms and responses to symptoms are inadequate, i.e. inadequate doses of analgesia and laxatives' (Dunlop and Hockley, 1990).

TEACHING NURSING STAFF TO CARE FOR THE DYING IN A BUSY GENERAL WARD

When teaching or advising nursing staff on general wards, it is necessary to gain the cooperation and assistance of the ward sister in explaining to junior staff the meaning of palliation in terminal care. According to the *Oxford Dictionary* the Latin *palliare* means 'to cloak'; it might be preferable to substitute the expression 'to shield' or 'to protect' in situations where there are distressing symptoms. Therefore palliation could also mean alleviation of the symptoms of the disease without curing it.

Once it has been established by the medical staff that no further investigations or curative treatment are advisable or applicable, the appropriate palliation is recommended. Nurses should be reminded that it is unnecessary to continue what have, in some wards, become automatically routine tasks known as:

- daily weights;
- 4-hourly TPR and BP;
- daily urine testing.

The medical notes often state: 'Keep comfortable – TLC'. Although the symptoms mentioned earlier are documented in detail elsewhere in this book, the following problems have been highlighted as of particular importance for nurses working in hospitals to recognize and understand.

Pain

This may be physical, emotional, social or spiritual. It is the physical pain that needs addressing first by locating the cause; is it related to:

- tumour site?
- bony metastases?
- chest pain?
- constipation?
- full bladder?
- nerve involvement?
- muscle spasm?
- headache?
- bony fracture?

The nursing care and management of these symptoms will depend on the outcome of good physical and medical examination and X-ray results which are of prime importance in diagnosis. For example, X-ray will determine pathological fracture and bony and lung metastases; abdominal X-ray and rectal examination will determine any faecal impaction. The use of a CT scan is a valuable diagnostic procedure for patients who complain of a continual headache accompanied by nausea; this may reveal cerebral metastases, the treatment for which would be high-dose glucocorticosteroids and sometimes palliative radiotherapy. Nurses need to be reminded that it is usual for high-dose glucocorticosteroids (e.g. dexamethasone 16 mg daily) to be prescribed to control headache due to raised intracranial pressure from cerebral metastases, which will not necessarily be relieved by conventional analgesia.

Having elicited the nature and the cause of the pain then the principles of the 'analgesic ladder' should be applied. Co-analgesics such as the non-steroidal anti-inflammatory drugs, antidepressants, antibiotics and gluco-corticosteroids, as mentioned above, may also help (Chapter 5).

Anorexia

Cancer cachexia, weight loss and dysphagia are very common in the patient dying of cancer. Before the hospital dietician is consulted, the nurse should carefully examine the patient's mouth with a torch which may reveal candidiasis (oral thrush), ulcers, ill-fitting dentures or other dental problems. The appropriate oral hygiene and mouth care should be instituted with a suitable mouthwash and/or the use of a soft toothbrush and toothpaste. These measures may help to improve the patient's swallowing and therefore their appreciation of small nutritional supplements such as the milk-based Build-up, Complan, Fresubin and Ensure or anything else that the patient fancies or enjoys. To stimulate an appetite an apéritif, such as sherry, may be given before meals. It is also psychologically more appropriate to present it in a suitable glass, as would happen in a social setting, rather than in a medicine cup.

Constipation

This is a common problem in the dying patient who takes analgesia such as co-proxamol, dihydrocodeine, morphine or diamorphine regularly. Lack of exercise and fluid intake will be added contributors to constipation. Good bowel management must be instituted immediately. A regular bowel softener and evacuant such as co-danthramer is prescribed. If there is gross faecal impaction a warm olive oil retention enema should be given slowly over a period of 10–15 minutes and retained overnight. The action of the warm oil will soften the hard faeces which may be expelled following a Microlax or soap and water enema the next morning. This procedure can be repeated daily until the bowel has been opened normally. Glycerine suppositories given rectally may be all that is required, but in severe cases a manual evacuation of faeces may be necessary.

Insomnia

Insomnia may be due to several reasons such as pain (emotional and spiritual) or hospital noise. Patients will not be used to sharing a bedroom with several others and may find it difficult to overcome the attendant irritations such as snoring and restlessness which are inevitable in a ward containing ill people. This is where the night nurses must be very sensitive to the needs of the dying patient; they may divulge all sorts of personal thoughts, fears and anxieties and the nurse should be prepared to listen and reassure the patient that they are not alone. Night tends to bring out the fear of the unknown and it should be regarded as a great privilege for the nurse to accompany a frightened patient through the small hours, long as they may seem. Sleep can usually follow after sensitively handled human interaction. The offer of a hot drink or a small tot of brandy in warm milk may work wonders. A change of position, a rearrangement of pillows and bedding are also helpful.

Many patients in hospital wards have had sleepless nights due to continuing activity. It is not only the stiffly starched aprons swishing past their beds, but the insensitive chatter; leather rather than rubber-soled shoes on the feet of night staff; incessant telephone bells and the rattle of trolleys that contribute to a disturbed night's sleep. It is worth remembering to switch the telephone to a soft ringing tone which can still be heard during the night hours. For dying patients unwanted noise causes friction in their minds. They do not have the energy to concentrate on important issues directly concerning themselves, let alone cope with unnecessary intrusions like blaring television sets displaying four different channels in the confined space of a hospital ward. Diplomacy on the part of the ward staff is essential in such a situation where there needs to be a reciprocal awareness of the needs of other patients who are in varying stages of disease. According to Florence Nightingale:

> Unnecessary noise or noise that creates expectation in the mind, is that which hurts the patient. Unnecessary noise then, is the most cruel absence of care which can be inflicted either on sick or well.
>
> (Baly, 1991)

Weakness and malaise

These will increase as bodily functions decrease and the patient will gradually be confined to bed and may feel hopeless and helpless. If this lethargy is due to anaemia a blood transfusion can improve the condition. The general feeling of well-being may be helped by a glucocorticosteroid (e.g. dexamethasone). At this stage, the debilitated patient, for whom everything is such an effort, will appreciate assistance with personal hygiene and mouth care. The luxury of an assisted, unhurried bath can promote a feeling of comforting relaxation and well-being.

Dyspnoea

Dyspnoea or breathlessness is a very frightening symptom and patients can be extremely demanding of nursing staff time. Nevertheless it is essential for the patient to know they are not alone with their fear. Simple nursing measures, such as moving the bed nearer an open window, provision of an electric fan or the removal of clutter and vases of flowers from the bed-table and locker, will help. To aid expansion of the lungs and to ease breathing, the patient may be settled in a sitting position extending the arms in front and resting them on raised pillows on the bed-table.

Medical treatment of breathlessness depends on the causes. These may include:

- anaemia – the patient may benefit from blood transfusion;
- congestive cardiac failure – may benefit from diuretics;
- chest infection – antibiotics may be prescribed;
- pleural effusion – a pleural tap will assist breathing. Lycoscine given subcutaneously or by syringe driver is usually recommended to ease this problem along with that of the death rattle. Gentle physiotherapy is occasionally given.

Whether the patient is dying from lung cancer or chronic obstructive airways disease, breathlessness and its attendant anxiety is often relieved, especially in the elderly, by a small dose of oral morphine (2.5–5 mg 4-hourly). It may also be given via a nebulizer and in this case oral morphine should continue for pain control. When all the above measures have been considered the use of oxygen is not usually necessary. An additional aid that may be adopted is the use of relaxation exercises and possibly the use of cassettes.

Nausea and vomiting

These are very unpleasant for the patient to endure but before treatment is started the cause must be established.

Causes of nausea and vomiting

- Anxiety and fear may be relieved by an anxiolytic drug such as diazepam. Referral to a counsellor or psychotherapist may also be beneficial if the patient is well enough. The nurses on the ward can help by continually reassuring the patient and encouraging breathing exercises for hyperventilators, methods of relaxation and diversional therapies.
- Raised intracranial pressure is caused by cerebral oedema. The recognized treatment for this is high-dose glucocorticosteroids such as dexamethasone 4 mg q.d.s. It is important that the last dose is given before 6 pm since it may be stimulant and so keep the patient awake at night.
- Hypercalcaemia is also common in terminal cancer. Patients may be confused, constipated and dehydrated. It may be wrongly assumed that the confusion is caused by opioids and if these are mistakenly reduced, more pain and anxiety can result. Hypercalcaemic patients will benefit from intravenous rehydration, one of the diphosphonate group of drugs such as pamidronate and treatment for constipation.
- Intestinal obstruction is a common complication in patients with advanced ovarian and colorectal cancer. Surgery to relieve the obstruction may be considered but in the dying patient conservative treatment is all that may be necessary so that the discomfort of passing nasogastric tubes can be avoided. The vomiting is often controlled by adding such drugs as haloperidol and cyclizine to a syringe driver. Metoclopramide should be avoided in the obstructed patient, as it promotes bowel peristalsis which may cause more pain and discomfort. Relief of constipation should be maintained (by the rectal route) since this may also be the cause of the vomiting. Obviously adequate mouth care must be maintained to avoid the horrid taste of faeculent vomit in the mouth.

- Gastric irritation due to carcinoma of the stomach may be relieved by metoclopramide given before meals. If there is gastric stasis because there is pressure on the stomach, due to an enlarged liver, pancreatic tumour or ascites, the condition of squashed stomach syndrome is diagnosed which may result in hiccoughs and can be most distressing. A defoaming agent such as dimethicone taken after meals may help.
- Radiotherapy and chemotherapy are other causes of vomiting. Patients travelling to a radiotherapy department should receive an antiemetic, such as Kwells (hyoscine 300 μg), prior to the journey. Chemotherapy, especially cisplatin, is a well-known cause of nausea and vomiting and patients may be given a combination of antiemetic, sedative and glucocorticosteroid prior to treatment, i.e. metoclopramide, lorazepam and dexamethasone. A new drug, ondansetron, is also proving effective.

Cough

Cough is extremely irritating and exhausting for the dying patient. If it is productive due to a chest infection, gentle physiotherapy and a broad spectrum antibiotic, such as chloramphenicol, may be prescribed. If the cough is dry, menthol steam inhalations and a codeine based linctus may help and should be given regularly.

Oedema

The limbs may be grossly oedematous due to obstruction of the lymphatic drainage system. Lymphoedema in the arms of women following mastectomy is unsightly. The physiotherapist can help by the application of intermittent compression sleeves to the limb which, if used regularly, will reduce the swelling. Abdominal ascites, causing distention and breathlessness, can easily be relieved by an abdominal paracentesis.

Sore mouth

The emphasis on good mouth care is maintained with all the previously mentioned symptoms. If the patient can use a toothbrush this is ideal but the nurse may have to intervene and use applicators for cleaning the mouth and applying agents such as Bonjela for sore gums. Oral and oesophageal thrush may be treated with nystatin mouthwash, Daktarin gel or fluconazole orally. Dentures should also be sterilized. Sores and ulcers, especially in patients who have received chemotherapy, may result in herpes on the lips, which can be remedied by topical acyclovir cream.

Agitation and confusion

Confusion and restlessness in the last 24 to 48 hours of life can be most distressing for the patient and their relatives. A nurse should examine the patient and check to see if they have a full bladder or other physical problems and deal with them immediately. Staying with the agitated patient, keeping the area quiet and subdued should help to reassure and calm them. Likewise having familiar objects and familiar people, such as the family and friends, around can also help alleviate restlessness. However, it may be necessary to commence a subcutaneous syringe driver with haloperidol and/or midazolam.

Dysphagia

Difficulty in swallowing is a common symptom of patients with advanced carcinoma of the oesophagus. Repeated dilatations to endoscopy or insertion of an oesophageal tube do help, but so often despite these measures these patients have lost a lot of weight and are very anorexic. They may still be able to swallow soft or liquidized foods such as Fresubin and Ensure. Because these symptoms have not been dealt with at home, these patients often have had to be admitted to hospital with progression of their disease and uncontrolled symptoms.

Measures to aid well-being

When nursing dying patients in the busy life of acute general wards it is the little details of nursing care that can make such a difference to their feeling of well-being – to patients and their relatives they become immensely important. For instance:

1. *Hair care* – For women this is their crowning glory. If the hospital hairdresser is not available provision for washing and setting by a nurse can be made and enjoyed by them both. For women who have had cytotoxic chemotherapy resulting in alopecia, a good wig well groomed and the daily changing of head scarves and turbans will not only enhance their appearance but will be a psychological boost to their morale. There should be provision of electric shavers for male patients; these are also more easily handled by nurses if the hospital barber is not available.
2. *Deafness* – This may be a problem in the elderly. Simply looking into the ears with an auriscope will ascertain whether the ear drum is blocked by wax. This can easily be relieved by the installation of Cerumol or sodium bicarbonate ear drops four times a day for a week followed by syringing of the ear. When normal hearing returns it

makes such a difference to the patient's ability to communicate with family and friends.

3. *Eyes* – Cataract operations in the elderly are a simple procedure for the ophthalmic surgeon and the improved eyesight can bring such renewed pleasure and delight to a weary patient. Cleaning an unwell patient's spectacles when they are tired and weak removes yet another burden and enhances their ability to see more clearly.
4. *Mouth and throat* – Oral hygiene has been dealt with in an earlier chapter. Some patients may experience halitosis – foul-smelling breath – from lung cancer and will need antibiotics to relieve the problem. If, however, this is due to oral cancers then meticulous mouth care is essential and the use of antibiotics such as metronidazole for anaerobic infections will be needed. The provision of favoured fruit sweets may also help. Ill-fitting dentures due to gum atrophy may give rise to embarrassment. A dental opinion should be sought to remedy this.

   Patients with tracheostomy are in special need of support and care. Communication can be most difficult and at times frightening for both patient and carer. The provision of bibs and clean dressings, blouse or shirt are essential for personal hygiene and dignity. A writing pad and pencil on which they can indicate their needs and wishes is essential, as well as a bell close at hand, which enables the patient to indicate the need for attention.
5. *Hands and feet* – Nails must be kept trimmed; manicure and pedicure are relaxing and enjoyable treatments. Chiropody is available in most hospital settings. Reflexology is a complementary therapy which can be explored with some patients who could find it not only relaxing but therapeutic.
6. *Fungating lesions* – These may be visible on breast tumour, on abdominal wall or elsewhere and have a foul odour which can be most distressing for the patient and family. There are many preparations available in hospital to obviate these odours, e.g. sprays and air fresheners, but for women in hospital a favourite perfume, clean night attire and scrupulously clean linen, changed immediately it is soiled or stained, is preferable. Men may be encouraged to use aftershave lotions. The use of aromatherapy essences and massage may also relieve the anxiety of the patient if they feel unclean. Also, if anaerobic infections are present, antibiotics will be useful.
7. *Apparatus* – Many dying patients have various tubes and pumps attached to their bodies such as syringe drivers, urinary catheters or gastrostomies. To maintain a sense of dignity for the patient it is possible for some equipment to be placed in halters or cotton bags at the side of the bed. If the patient is mobile, however, it is much nicer for them to have this equipment in a pocket or pouch, so that their hands are free.

COMING TO TERMS WITH DEATH AND DYING AND TEACHING OTHERS

It is not until distressing symptoms are under control that we can begin to talk and listen to patients about how they feel, what they understand about their illness, what the doctor has said to them and their understanding of why they are feeling the way they do. 'Coming to terms' may be a painful and stressful reality in that they are not going to get better. One of the main complaints of relatives is the lack of communication in hospital: 'Poor communication can cause more suffering than many of the symptoms of terminal disease' (Gooch, 1988).

Hospital nurses still find it difficult to come to terms with giving bad news or even expanding on what is already rather obvious, due to their own feelings of inadequacy and helplessness. For example, a dying patient was surrounded by his family who were quietly reading and knitting while keeping their vigil, as they had done for the past 24 hours; they had no idea that his breathing had altered; the colour in his face was draining and his extremities were cold and blue. No-one had told them that he was going to die very soon, possibly within the next hour, until they were informed very suddenly and had to make hasty goodbyes. This could have been less distressing for all concerned if the changes in respiration rate and pallor had been observed more closely and the family had also been kept in touch with what these indicated in terms of the patient's approaching demise. In situations like this the giving of information promptly is crucial for the relatives so that they are able to accept what is happening preparatory to coping with the bereavement period.

The skills of communication need to be addressed by all involved in the care of the dying patient and their family. These include medical and nursing staff, physiotherapists, occupational therapists, social workers, chaplains, nursing auxiliaries and domestic staff. Good communication depends on the personality of the communicator and not necessarily on their professional status.

The responsibility of communicating the diagnosis and the significance of changes which take place in the varying stages of advancing disease must lie with the doctor and senior nurses. They need, therefore, to be familiar with the results of recent investigations and have the knowledge to interpret them to the patient and their family. Time may be at a premium for the patient and ideally the doctor and nurse should be together when information is imparted so that a team approach is adopted in caring for the patient and their family.

In the hospital setting it is often difficult to find privacy in which this kind of meeting can take place; ideally an office should be available with an 'engaged' notice on the door, bleeps and telephone lines turned off and staff advised not to interrupt. An hour or more may have to be set aside for this meeting as it may be crucial. The whole family, together with listening professionals, will have the opportunity to explore, with honesty and hope, the various goals to be met and develop the kinds of strategies and coping mechanisms that can be helpful within the time that is left. This time is also beneficial in planning for the bereavement to come. How often have we heard from the bereaved, 'If only I'd known earlier we could have done so much more together'. Feelings of guilt and anger at things left unsaid and undone live with bereaved relatives for a long time.

When starting a conversation with a patient suffering from a life-threatening disease and their family, it is advisable to find out what they already know and understand and what they really want to know. To do this it helps to start from the beginning of the illness, go through the results of the scans, tests, biopsies and so on and follow their treatment such as surgery, radiotherapy or chemotherapy. This is time consuming work and demands every ounce of listening ability to discern what the patient really thinks and feels. This need not be an interrogative exercise and must be geared to how ill or frail the patient may be. Gradually the patient will understand what you are saying and may say:

'Thank you for being so honest'
or 'I know I'm not getting better'
or 'I know it's a matter of time'
or 'Now I can get on with . . .'
or 'How long have I got?'

These sentiments have been expressed in an excellent video recording 'The Cancer Journey' by Dr Sheila Cassidy and is strongly recommended to every medical and nursing college for teaching purposes. Dr Robert Buckman, in his book *I Don't Know What to Say*, advises his medical students to practise interview techniques with each other, as '. . . breaking bad news is not a divine gift but a skilled technique which has to be learnt' (Buckman, 1989).

We as nurses must persevere both in learning for ourselves and teaching others the art and skill of communicating with the dying; ideally this should be given high priority in each ward's teaching programme. As staff become more confident in this aspect of caring for the dying, they should be encouraged to broaden and deepen their exploration of this skill.

Most hospitals have a chaplaincy team. They should be informed if the patient expresses the wish to be visited (or to see their own spiritual advisor) to offer the ministry of healing or anointing of the sick or to receive other sacraments. Spiritual pain in the dying patient may be a real burden and cause sleepless nights and agitated days. It may be a simple act of absolution by the priest that is needed or the sharing of a long-standing and hitherto repressed grievance which the patient is seeking to resolve with someone who has become aware of that need. This may well be the nurse.

> An aware person has something to communicate to others from the depths of their being.
>
> (Riem, 1993)

> A person who is not afraid to wait in darkness before God will be more able to avoid erecting defences against the pain of another's darkness or the stench of another's physical decay; she will not succumb to parentalism, an infrangible cheerfulness, the tendency to chatter . . . his fearlessness will provide an atmosphere in which the patient will feel able to abandon some of his own defences, and his humility will open their meeting to truth.
>
> (Riem, 1993)

As we live in a multiracial society it would be expedient to examine our understanding of the various cultural rituals practised by people of differing races and religions. Sometimes it is necessary to employ interpreters to assist in our communications. Rabbi Julia Neuberger's book *Caring for Dying People of Different Faiths* (1987) gives details of how to care, both physically and spiritually, for patients from the ancient religions of the East, Sikhism, Hinduism, Islam and Buddhism, and also Christianity and Judaism.

It is obviously a priority to be aware of the needs of someone who cannot communicate in English. This is where the reassurance of touch or the warmth of a smile can release tensions and fear.

Psychological care of the dying has been well documented by Peter Maguire (1985). He describes '. . . distancing tactics by doctors and nurses unable to get close to patients ensuring their own emotional safety' and these self-defence strategies obviate any sensitivity to awareness of the needs of the dying that is so crucial to good terminal care.

> Are we as nurses prepared to get close to those who are dying, to allow them to tell us what they know, what they want to know and have we the courage to stay and share?
>
> (Ainsworth-Smith and Speck, 1982)

TEACHING RELATIVES HOW TO CONTINUE CARE AT HOME

Before a dying patient is discharged for home care, it is essential that all the services to be involved are informed and prepared to receive the patient. This may sometimes take up to a week to ten days depending on the home circumstances. Planned hospital discharge, therefore, is vital and may include an assessment and home visit by the occupational therapist. It may be necessary to provide rails on the stairs and in the bathroom, a raised toilet seat or a commode or urinal. Special bedding or even a hospital bed may be necessary. Pressure relieving mattresses such as a Spenco or an electrically controlled inflatable mattress such as a Nimbus or Pegasus may be required. Provision of a 'monkey-pole' will enable the patient to lift themselves in bed and extra pillows may provide more comfort.

For patients with tracheostomies, oxygen cylinders can be ordered by the GP through the local chemist. The GP, district nurses and Macmillan nurses must be willing to take on this responsibility and all efforts made to procure the necessary equipment. It may also be necessary for the physiotherapist to be involved. A Marie Curie night nursing service is available to relieve the family, allowing them to sleep. Ambulance transport must be booked and they will require information as to the location of the dwelling; if it is above ground-floor level, where there is no lift, at least a two-man crew with either a carrying chair or stretcher will be needed.

On leaving the hospital the relatives must be given at least a week's supply of any drugs, dressings, incontinence pads and mouth care equipment needed. They should be taught how to turn and lift the patient and change the sheets in a manner that is comfortable for the patient. They can also be shown how to change a syringe driver if they wish to take on this responsibility. The district nurse will prepare the solution daily.

CARING FOR THE ELDERLY WHO ARE DYING IN HOSPITAL

The principles of earlier discussions remain the same. Patients dying of old age in geriatric wards may have no relatives at all. Therefore the prospect of going home is not practical. Patients dying from cerebrovascular disease may need long term care in a nursing home for the elderly. Great sensitivity is needed in nursing these patients; they may have impaired hearing and sight and may be unable to feed themselves or communicate verbally. Nurses should monitor the serving of food, for instance, so that it is presented as attractively as possible and at the right temperature.

The introduction of activities which divert their attention from the immediate environment and stimulate their interests, thereby improving their quality of life, can be introduced onto the ward. If long term memory recall can be stimulated by simple activities such as an Old Time Music Hall 'sing-along', organized, perhaps, by volunteer helpers, it may produce a wealth of information which if observed may be an aid to ways of enhancing nursing care. It is therefore essential that nursing staff encourage relatives or helpers to join in the process of stimulating these patients so that observation of their responses can be a source of information which nurses can use in meeting their needs.

Many elderly patients dying in hospital will die from pneumonia which will require good nursing care. The dying patient and their bond with the family can be seen to have its parallel in the geriatric ward which for some has been a home. On the demise of any long-stay patient there may be for some other patients with sufficient awareness a sense of loss and grief similar to the family situation; this, too, needs to be met. The discerning nurse will be sensitive to such needs.

CARING FOR THE DYING PATIENT IN THE INTENSIVE THERAPY UNIT (ITU)

> Intensive therapy units are structurally designed for a specific purpose, to maintain life through acute but temporary life-threatening episodes.
>
> (Daly, 1990)

Nursing staff caring for patients in ITU have many problems with which to come to terms:

- The patients are often very young people; they may have had road traffic accidents or injuries resulting from terrorist attacks.
- Staff work under great pressure to cure the patient and death feels like failure.
- Death may occur soon after admission and the family will be very shocked.
- They will be surrounded by several patients who are seriously ill requiring intensive nursing and medical care.

Obviously there needs to be tremendous team work in caring for these patients and their families. Support groups are essential for the welfare and well-being of staff because of the incredible pressures put upon them.

> A good death involves individual perceptions and interpretations of the living/dying process, as well as shared observations of the event of death. It is most likely to be defined as 'good' when it reflects an individual's way of living. An individual's usual way of living is difficult to observe in the ITU, a factor that contributes to seeing death as separate from life.
>
> (Daly, 1990)

CARING FOR THE TERMINALLY ILL PATIENT WITH RENAL DISEASE

These patients will be well known to the staff in the renal dialysis unit. They will have undergone treatment over months or years and may have had renal transplant surgery. Decisions will have been made to abandon dialysis or surgery and the patient, watched by their relatives, will die after years of treatment. The principles already described still apply in the nursing care. Special diets are now unimportant and the patient may have anything they fancy. Empty catheter drainage bags will be the result of non-functioning kidneys. Constant skin irritation and involuntary twitching due to uraemia are extremely distressing and therefore palliation of these symptoms is necessary. Sedation with diazepam and the application of topical creams such as Eurax may help.

Staff support groups are necessary in this specialized area and it may be necessary to employ an outside facilitator.

DEATH IN THE ACCIDENT AND EMERGENCY (A & E) DEPARTMENT

Death in the accident and emergency department is usually traumatic because it is often sudden and so unexpected. The patient may be admitted in shock and the relatives are shocked by the news of the sudden admission. Admission to an A & E department is usually due to a medical or surgical crisis like a heart attack or trauma such as those caused by road traffic accidents or domestic incidents. The A & E department is not usually the place for people dying from known malignant disease; provision should have been made for their management either at home or in a hospice.

Shalley and Cross (1984) state that the majority of patients they studied in an East Birmingham hospital who died did so from medical emergencies such as myocardial infarction, cerebrovascular accidents, chronic obstructive airways disease and bronchopneumonia in the elderly. Half of the patients they studied were between 70 and 80 years old. Common also were the infant infections such as purulent meningitis and sudden infant death syndrome in babies under 12 months. Patients admitted to A & E with surgical problems were much fewer in number and were mainly men with ruptured aortic aneurysms. Other surgical emergencies were gastro-intestinal bleeding due to peptic ulceration and infections causing peritonitis. The traumatic admissions were mainly young people involved in road traffic accidents sustaining severe head and chest injuries.

It would therefore seem that the majority of patients admitted in shock to an A & E department were found to have a diagnosis of a medical rather than a surgical nature. Shalley and Cross's recommendations were for improved training of doctors together with access to more and better facilities in medical emergency training programmes. They also emphasized that the crucial period between admission to hospital and obtaining specialist opinion must be better catered for in medical A & E training.

As far as the nurses are concerned in A & E, care must be devoted to the family. They should be kept informed of what is happening in the resuscitation area and if they wish to remain with their relative every provision should be made, as far as is practical, to meet their request even though the situation may be very traumatic for them. They need to be informed of the changes of condition which take place in the patient; what the various machines are for and if finally the patient dies they need to have this explained clearly in language they understand.

In our multiracial society it is often the young English-speaking child who is sent for to interpret what is being said about their relative. A & E departments should have access to interpreters, social workers, chaplains and health visitors. If a patient's relatives do not have a telephone it is usually a police officer who undertakes to inform them.

As has already been stated, 'Poor communication can create more suffering than many of the symptoms of terminal disease' (Gooch, 1988) and this statement is confirmed by the findings of a study in Lancashire (McGuinness, 1986). Informing relatives was not observed to be a priority in this study; this conclusion was drawn from the fact that nurses spent only about ten minutes when informing relatives of a death. The doctor spent even less time, about three minutes, in explaining the outcome of the resuscitation procedure. Clearly time is precious, but time given to the family is well spent for it may avoid psychological trauma in the bereavement period, as outlined by Parkes (1982).

Many patients with cardiac emergencies are brought in dead as attempts at resuscitation in the ambulance have been unsuccessful. This can be a traumatic experience for the staff as well as for relatives of the deceased. In the confusion that may follow it is the nurse's duty to be sensitive and ensure that the person identifying the body is the most reliable source of information concerning the deceased. In accident cases features can be so disfigured that it is almost impossible to give an identification.

SUDDEN DEATH

To enable nurses to handle sudden death situations, up-to-date knowledge of resuscitation procedures is essential and should be continually reappraised.

In these days of transplant surgery and organ donation the medical and nursing team need to be sensitive in their approach to the relatives when seeking permission to remove parts of the body, even if the adult patient carries a donor card. It must be remembered, however, that the coroner must be informed of the patient's death if it was:

- within 24 hours of admission to hospital;
- within 24 hours of surgery;
- death following a road traffic accident;
- a sudden, unexpected death in hospital.

In an article on sudden infant deaths, McGuinness (1986) states that parents should be allowed to hold their dead babies and dress them in the clothes normally worn so that a photograph may be taken, preferably with an Instamatic camera. A photograph of the baby will allow them, in their bereavement, to have real proof of the child having existed and memories of their features. The department which may come into contact with infants, that is maternity, A & E or the children's ward, should have access to a Polaroid camera.

> In a profession of carers and supporters it is important to keep matters in perspective. The grief belongs to the relatives; the nurse's role is to facilitate the grieving process. Nurses cannot bear this pain for them. It is possible to take a professional pride in getting such a difficult job well done.
>
> (Burgess, 1992)

Suicide

It may not be generally known that until 1961 suicide was a criminal offence since it was considered to be self-murder. Generally it is unexpected, although in hindsight families may recall the expression of feelings of depression and other such negative emotions by the patient.

Dealing with bereaved relatives of a successful suicide who has been brought into hospital will possibly be more complex for the nurse; there will not only be the usual emotions expressed by the bereaved but a more reinforced sense of guilt and feeling of responsibility that the cause of death has evoked. Acceptance of the death of a loved one is painful enough: death brought about in an unnatural way, deliberately self-inflicted, must be even more difficult to accept.

This will be most upsetting for the relatives or those closest to the victim and the nurse will need to encourage them to talk, express their feelings and reassure them that they could not have prevented the tragedy, thereby alleviating the sense of responsibility. They will, of course, need long term bereavement support involving other agencies which, if at all possible, the hospital should help to locate.

An American study by Farmer (1984) found that there were 56 self-destructive behaviours leading to suicide. One included the refusal to continue with chemotherapy and radiotherapy. This must surely create a dilemma for oncology nurses but they can only support and guide and help their patients to cope.

In the general hospital we are, sadly, only too aware of the weekend overdoses of paracetamol by people who, because of many socioeconomic problems, find life today very depressing and unfulfilling. It is these cries for help with which the nurse on the general ward is confronted. These patients may be in beds alongside dying patients for whom the prospect of living would be a wonderful miracle for them and their families. It is a most difficult dichotomy for the nurse but it has to be dealt with impartially and the resources found to treat the victim with psychological help, compassion and understanding.

THE PATIENT DYING WITH NON-MALIGNANT DISEASE

It is sometimes said that patients who are dying from cancer or motor neurone disease are in a fortunate position in that they have access to hospice care, whereas patients dying from chronic, long term, debilitating illness do not. Patients suffering from senile dementia, Alzheimer's disease, multiple sclerosis, Parkinson's disease and chronic respiratory illnesses will require long term nursing care which may be at home or in an institution such as a nursing home or a geriatric ward. Whether confined to bed or wheelchair, these patients will require the nursing care described in this chapter. They should have all the resources available to assist them in their daily activities such as occupational therapy, speech therapy, physiotherapy, tissue viability assessment, nutritional advice and the continence service.

The GP and the community nursing service have the task of not only caring for the patient but also for the relative who carries the brunt of the care. Facilities must be made available for respite care in hospital or other institution, as well as day hospital provision, enabling the relative to have a break. Most relatives will have feelings of guilt about letting go of their loved one for this purpose, but careful and tactful persuasion to allow this to happen does relieve tiredness, which the burden of constant caring brings about, and enables them to continue to care, feeling refreshed.

If, however, the patient becomes too dependent on the carers at home because they may be unconscious or physically too heavy, longer term hospital admission may then be sought. The relatives may wish to continue with their care and may offer to do so in the hospital setting with the back-up of professional staff and equipment. Some hospital wards may welcome offers of this help.

CONCLUSION

Dr Sheila Cassidy, in the introduction to her book *Sharing the Darkness – The Spirituality of Caring*, says:

> We professionals have expensive ring-side seats at the fight: and we have a close-up view of the players who are stripped of sophistication and pretence . . .

So we are very privileged to be allowed to be close and intimately involved with those who are finishing their journeys in our care. This is surely a challenge to enable us to live up to our vocational calling.

REFERENCES

Ainsworth-Smith, I. and Speck, P. (1982) *Letting Go*, SPCK, London.

Baly, M. (1991) *'As Miss Nightingale Said . . .': Florence Nightingale through her Sayings, A Victorian Perspective*, Scutari, London, p. 65.

Buckman, R. (1989) *I Don't Know What to Say. How to Help and Support Someone who is Dying*, Papermac, London, p. 3.

Burgess, K. (1992) Supporting bereaved relatives in A & E. *Nursing Standard*, **6**(19), 36–40.

Cassidy, S. (1988) *Sharing the Darkness – The Spirituality of Caring*, Darton, Longman and Todd, London.

Daly, B.J. (ed.) (1990) *ITU Nursing*, Medical Examination Publishing, London.

Dunlop, R.J. and Hockley, J.M. (1990) *Terminal Care Support Teams, The Hospital–Hospice Interface*, Oxford Medical Publications, Oxford, p. 7.

Farmer, L.M. (1984) *Suiciding in Cancer Patients, Implications for Nursing*, Paper presented at the International Cancer Nursing Conference, Australia.

Gooch, J. (1988) Dying in the ward. *Nursing Times*, **84**(21), 38–9.

Macguire, P. (1985) Barriers to psychological care of the dying (distancing tactics). *British Medical Journal*, **291**, 1711–13.

McGuinness, S. (1986) Coping with death. *Nursing Times*, **82**(12), 28–31.

Neuberger, J. (1987) *Caring for Dying People of Different Faiths*, The Lisa Sainsbury Foundation Series, Austen Cornish, London.

Office of Population Census and Surveys (1980) *Mortality Statistics for 1978, England and Wales*, HMSO, London.

Parkes, C.M. (1982) *Bereavement – Studies of Grief in Adult Life*, Penguin, Harmondsworth.

Riem, R. (1993) Stronger than dead – *A Study of Love for the Dying*, Darton, Longman and Todd, London, p. 29.

Shalley, M.J. and Cross, A.B. (1984) Which patients are likely to die in an A & E department? *British Medical Journal*, **289**(6442), 419–421.

FURTHER READING

Baines, M. (1984) Control of other symptoms, in *Management of the Terminal Malignant Disease*, 2nd edn, (ed. C. Saunders), Edward Arnold, London, p. 100.

Cassidy, S. (1986) Emotional distress in terminal cancer – a discussion paper. *Journal of the Royal Society of Medicine*, **79**, p. 717.

Hector, W. and Whitfield, S. (1982) *Nursing Care for the Dying Patient and the Family*, Heinemann Medical, London.

Care in a hospice

18

INTRODUCTION

Members of the public have perhaps the clearest understanding of the meaning or expectation of 'care in a hospice'. To be worthy of the title 'hospice', the care is expected to be of a high quality. The new hospice movement has tended to be synonymous with 'terminal care for cancer patients'. More recently, since the Royal College of Physicians has recognized this new speciality, the term 'palliative care' has emerged.

DEFINITION

The National Council for Hospice and Specialist Palliative Care Services (1993) has endorsed the definition used within the speciality, agreeing that palliative care (or terminal care) is the active, total care of patients whose disease process will no longer respond to curative intervention and treatment and for whom the goal must be the best quality of life for them and their families. Dame Cicely Saunders would resonate with this view as she has repeatedly claimed that a hospice is not a building but an attitude. It is this caring attitude that is one of the distinctive marks of a hospice.

BUILDINGS

When providing an inpatient service, however, the building cannot be ignored. In keeping with a philosophy of care, planning committees, along with their architects and builders, expend much time and energy in designing the most attractive premises that are financially viable. With imagination and skill, older buildings can be upgraded. Good use of materials and colour can transform the interior decoration. The use of landscaping which allows ponds, fountains or waterfalls can be restful and uplifting. Attention needs to be given to the view from beds and sitting areas. City dwellers may appreciate seeing the passing traffic and perhaps spotting their usual bus while others may favour being surrounded by beautiful natural scenery.

There is a continuing debate on the ideal size of wards, either the traditional four-bedded or the provision of single rooms. As pointed out by Seale (1989), it is not usual for a hospice to routinely move a dying patient into a single room as it can produce feelings of isolation and fear. Each ward or room, if not ensuite, needs toileting facilities nearby. The hospice shop, tea bar or restaurant can be a real lifesaver to visiting relatives and friends.

WELCOME

Another aspect of the caring attitude is expressed through the welcome accorded to everyone. Hospices tend to be small units, varying from 2–62 beds as stated in the *Directory of Hospice Services* (Hospice Information Service, 1993a). Due to their size it is possible to create a friendly, village-type atmosphere. The welcome of each new patient is given special priority. It is the usual practice to have a designated nurse to meet the patient on arrival for admission. The allocated person may be the primary nurse, team leader, ward sister or matron. While the patient is greeted and escorted to the ward the accompanying relative is being comforted as well. First impressions do count and time spent at this stage may well relieve and eliminate many future anxieties.

FAMILY CARE

Taking special care of the spouses of patients and including the family in the caring team has been observed by Parkes and Parkes (1984) as a hallmark of good hospice care. When relatives and the patient are at the centre of the care the hospice can be said to be functioning well. This appears to be more difficult to achieve in a larger hospital setting.

CHANGES

There are concerns among some hospice workers that routinization may be established within hospices as they grow in size and become more professional. This is partly influenced by the changes within the National Health Service. To keep abreast of these demands and innovations and to avoid being swamped by them, hospices have to adopt a more bureaucratic approach.

QUALITY AND STANDARDS

Until Help the Hospices formed the National Council for Hospice and Specialist Palliative Care Service each unit was very much on its own. Back in the mid-1980s Fenell (1985) recognized the need for a national organization in the New Zealand scene. He identified the need for a representative body to negotiate with government as well as offer other support. In this country the National Council has issued an occasional paper on *Quality, Standards, Organizational and Clinical Audit for Hospice and Palliative Care Services* (1992). Local working parties and committees are being formed to help hospice staff adjust to these changes. The hospice movement, according to James and Field (1992), could be described as being 'reformist'. Now these units have themselves to adjust to an outside influence.

Each hospice foundation aims to give a high quality of care but due to financial restraints, research and evaluation have been kept to a minimum. With the directives from the mainstream health service, that position is being reversed. Again James and Field (1992) point out that hospices, by virtue of their roles, were critics of the standards of terminal care within hospitals and elsewhere. If hospices now appear to be in close collaboration with their health service colleagues, they do so having achieved the ability to model good palliative care. Major progress has been made in symptom control and the ability to openly discuss prognosis with patients. The carers and staff have benefited from this openness.

SPIRITUAL CARE

According to Parkes and Parkes (1984) there is a more positive and active spiritual element in hospices than in other settings. James and Field (1992) also refer to the spiritual underpinning to be found within hospices. This can also be demonstrated by a genuine commitment to teamwork, where each person is listened to and can make a valuable contribution. When teams are cohesive and performing in this manner they are truly carrying on the tradition handed down by their charismatic founders.

HISTORY OF THE HOSPICE MOVEMENT

While the new hospice movement is dated from 1967 the word 'hospice' has its origins in the Roman word *hospes* – meaning both a host and a guest. From this tradition of hospitality, both hospitals for treatment of the sick and hospices for giving temporary help and accommodation can be traced back to the ancient world, but the dominant influence in the growth of hospices was Christianity (although the two concepts were interchangeable for several centuries).

Most of the credit for early hospices must be attributed to the Knights Hospitallers of the Order of St John of Jerusalem. These were founded in Malta in 1065, primarily for the task of caring for the sick and dying on pilgrimage to and from the Holy Land.

At the peak of their flowering, records show an attitude of great consideration and respect for the needs of the individual – what would be called today a holistic approach to care. The same was true of the medieval hospices operating throughout Europe; 750 were in existence in England alone.

Following the suppression of the monasteries and the dispersal of religious men and women, the sick, poor and dying were left without help and medicine and nursing remained at a low ebb for a considerable time, hospitals at that period being places to be dreaded and avoided at all costs.

It was not until the middle of the nineteenth century that the old idea of the hospice began to revive. The Sisters of Charity, founded by Vincent de Paul in 1600, had worked quietly for three centuries among the poorest and most despised members of French society and during the nineteenth century influenced such pioneers as the Protestant pastor Fliedner (who founded Kaiserswerth), Florence Nightingale and Elizabeth Fry.

In 1840 an Irishwoman, Mary Aikenhead, opened in Dublin a place of shelter and care for the dying and called it by the old medieval name of 'hospice'. She founded a new Apostolic order, the Religious Sisters of Charity, who in 1905 opened a similar house in London – St Joseph's Hospice – which has continued until the present day in caring for dying patients and those with chronic illnesses. Just before the opening of St Joseph's Hospice, two other hospices had opened in London – St Luke's, founded in 1894 by a Methodist minister, Mr Barrett, has been rebuilt and is known as Hereford Lodge. The other hospice, the Hostel of God, was started by a community of Anglican sisters. This closed for some years but is now operating under lay management and has been renamed Trinity Hospice.

While this development was proceeding in Europe, a parallel revival of the old hospice idea was taking place in America, through the work of a Dominican order of Sisters founded by Rose Hawthorne. Their first hospice opened in New York in 1899 and was followed by others. In the 1950s an important development was the establishment of the Marie Curie Foundation, which aimed to relieve the distress of patients dying with cancer and the strain on their families. Homes were set up to provide hospice care.

The highest point of the new hospice movement has been achieved through the work of Dame Cicely Saunders. In revolutionizing the approach to the control of pain and other distressing symptoms in dying patients and in re-emphasizing the right of the patient to a peaceful and dignified death, she has led the way and inspired others to introduce hospice care all over this country and on a worldwide basis.

At St Joseph's, where she was appointed fulltime medical officer and began her special work for dying patients, she was able to build on the tradition and practice of loving care carried out for more than half a century by this Christian community, whose original priority had been relieving the distress caused by widespread tuberculosis. In founding St Christopher's Hospice, the threads of care were traced back over nearly 2000 years and enriched with a new emphasis on scientific research and teaching.

THE WAY FORWARD

As with any movement or aspect of daily life the dilemma can arise of what to preserve from the long and valued tradition of the past and what to shed to enable a better future to emerge.

A proliferation of services sprang up during the 1970s and 1980s. Even though some leading hospice enthusiasts had called for a halt on new projects, local people continued to campaign for their own area. In the United Kingdom and Ireland the *Directory of Hospice Services* (Hospice Information Service, 1993a) shows that there are 193 inpatient units giving a total of 2993 beds. There are also 400 home and hospital based services and 200 day hospices. Some 25 new projects are in the planning stages. Helen House, Oxford, was the first hospice in the world founded exclusively for children (1982). There are now several others.

To meet the differing needs of people it could be argued that a variety of services are required to offer some element of choice. How to achieve this flexibility is part of the challenge of this decade.

Many people involved in palliative care have been concerned and puzzled as to why such a small proportion of patients from minority faiths and ethnic groups actually seek hospice admission. A new project is being launched with a view to improving their access to these services. This is another initiative of the National Council for Hospice and Specialist Palliative Care as advertised in the *Hospice Bulletin* (Hospice Information Service, 1993b).

While there is general agreement on endeavouring to reach all those in need of palliative care and to offer good holistic care through a teamwork model of care, a new debate has arisen regarding the narrow focus of hospice services. No one disputes that the dying will always be with us and that they deserve the best possible care. However, many ask if this knowledge and expertise should be confined to the group who are dying of cancer. Traditionally hospices have reserved a small percentage of beds for patients with such conditions as motor neurone disease or multiple sclerosis. The question remains, could hospices admit a wider group of patients and still maintain the other aspects of their philosophy which are apparently so appreciated by the public they serve?

The above questions have to be addressed within the hospice structure and with their supportive charities, the Marie Curie Cancer Care, the Sue Ryder Foundation, the Cancer Relief Macmillan Fund, not forgetting the influence and directives of the National Health Service. As fundamental issues are debated, those with managerial responsibilities need to be acutely aware of the potential recipients of their services. What Klagsburn (1981) stated is still true today: although a hospice need not be a religious organization, it would seem essential that there is a spiritual dimension to its structure – to the rational human being, suffering and death ultimately have to make sense in order for the person to remain human.

VALUE OF VOLUNTEERS

Volunteers are used extensively in hospices throughout the UK and elsewhere. They work in collaboration with the professional staff in promoting and sustaining the caring community which lies at the heart of hospice care at a time when modern health care tends to stress technology and cost-effectiveness. By giving their time, energy and skills freely, volunteers challenge the pragmatic values that are part of an ever-increasing businesslike culture that is slowly creeping into the hospice world.

The resources that volunteers make available are limitless. However, what they contribute to the spirit of hospices is by far their greatest gift.

Volunteers can play a key role in keeping the spirituality of the founding members of hospices alive. They help to maintain a warm, informal, caring atmosphere because they are not caught up in bureaucracy or stifled by regulations. They are less task oriented and more person centred. They are completely flexible about the amount of time spent with any particular person.

Volunteers are linked into and are involved in a network of relationships, not just within a hospice but in the wider community, thereby bonding staff, patients, relatives and friends into a community. It would be difficult to demonstrate the value of the contribution made by volunteers in terms of return on investment but the core of hospice care is friendship and hospitality and the presence of volunteers helps to keep that spirit alive at a time when hospices are experiencing pressure to adopt a more commercial approach.

Volunteers should never be considered or used as cheap labour or as substitutes for paid staff. Exploiting volunteers in this way undermines the spirit and value of their contribution. They should complement paid staff and work in partnership with them, thereby contributing a dimension to hospice care which might be difficult or impossible to achieve in a purely nurse/medical oriented environment.

The activities of the volunteers are as varied as the volunteers themselves – hairdressing, manicuring, complementary therapies, outings and befriending, hostessing and photography are just some of the ways in which volunteers can enhance the care given by the professionals, i.e. paid staff. But what we do for people is only one aspect of caring. There are times when just 'being with' someone is what is important. Sometimes patients or their relatives want someone to be with them, not to have to make conversation but merely to know that someone is there. It is in these situations that volunteers are 'manna from Heaven' and come into their own.

Ultimately the value of volunteers can only be fully realized by a disciplined voluntary service directed by a coordinator who should embody the spirit of the hospice and recognize the individual personalities and skills of volunteers and how to place them to their best advantage.

'Tailor-made' volunteers are a rarity so initial training and education are essential, as well as continual information. Coordinators also need support, guidance and training. There are some excellent organizations and networks within the United Kingdom and elsewhere which provide information packs and organize courses, etc. both for volunteers and coordinators which can enable a voluntary service to be professional and at the same time help to keep the spirituality of hospice care alive.

REFERENCES

Fennell, F.V. (1985) New horizons on the hospice scene. *New Zealand Nursing Journal*, **78**(10), 26–7.

Hospice Information Service (1993a) *Directory of Hospice Services*, St Christopher's Hospice, London.

Hospice Information Service (1993b) *Hospice Bulletin*, No. 19(3), St Christopher's Hospice, London.

James, N. and Field, D. (1992) The routinization of hospice: charisma and bureaucratization. *Social Science Medicine*, **34**(12), 1363–75.

Klagsburn, S.C. (1981) Hospice – a developing role, in *Hospice: The Living Idea*, (eds C.M. Saunders *et al.*), Edward Arnold, London.

National Council for Hospice and Specialist Palliative Care Services (1992)

Quality, Standards, Organizational and Clinical Audit for Hospice and Palliative Care Services, Occasional Paper No. 2, NCHSPCS, London.

National Council for Hospice and Specialist Palliative Care Services (1993) *Care in the Community for People who are Terminally Ill*, NCHSPCS, London, pp. 1–4.

Parkes, C.M. and Parkes, J. (1984) 'Hospice' versus 'hospital' care – re-evaluation after 10 years as seen by surviving spouses. *Postgraduate Medical Journal*, **60**, 120–4.

Seale, C.F. (1989) What happens in hospices: a review of research evidence. *Social Science Medicine*, **28**(6), 551–9.

FURTHER READING

Berzoni, L., Singer, D., Wray, Z. and Hutchinson, R. (1991) *Voluntary Services Coordinators in the National Health Service*, Advance Publishers.

Marteau, L. (1991) *A Vision of Life*, Bounty Services, Diss.

Sisters of Charity Health Service Council (1992) *Mission Effectiveness: The Mission Continues*, Sisters of Charity, New South Wales, Australia.

The place of complementary therapies

19

> We have learnt as a result of literally hundreds of experiments that there is a limit to the effectiveness of any given therapy but happily the effect of two or more therapies given in combination are cumulative.
>
> (Melzack and Wall, 1988)

Complementary therapies are frequently being used alongside conventional medicine in the care of the terminally ill patient. The diagnosis of cancer is not always as horrific as it seems in that people who have 'incurable cancer' actually 'live' with it. By accepting other therapies alongside acceptable medical treatments their quality of life can be greatly improved. There are many examples of complementary therapies. In this chapter we will highlight some of those most commonly used in which we, as aromatherapist, physiotherapist and nurse, have witnessed some beneficial results at Garden House Hospice where we all work.

Hospices today offer day care and respite care for patients and carers and give enormous support.

RELAXATION AND VISUALIZATION

There are many types of relaxation techniques including distraction, guided imagery and visualization.

Relaxation has been found to be beneficial in reducing a patient's pain levels and also in reducing stress levels. It is known to be beneficial to the immune system. Relaxation techniques are often taught in pain control clinics as a way of changing the body's response to pain.

In *Cash's Textbook of General Medicine and Surgical Conditions for Physiotherapists* (Downie, 1984) stress is described as 'a body's condition in which the physiology is set ready for activity'. Stress may be considered as a state of being threatened in any form. Thus a terminally ill patient may be feeling threatened by the illness, the consequences of the illness, alterations in lifestyle, learning to depend on others and/or approaching death. For the family, their loved one's illness, the caring for them and the consequences of the inevitable death of their loved one all cause great stress. It may also be provoking feelings of guilt, anger, denial and helplessness.

When a person is under stress their body reacts by the pituitary gland secreting adrenocorticotrophic hormone (ACTH) into the blood stream. This stimulates the thyroid gland to release thyroxine and the medullae of the adrenal gland releases adrenaline and noradrenaline. The release of these hormones results in numerous changes in the body, including increases in: heart action and blood pressure; metabolism of all cells; CO_2 in blood; respiratory rate; sweating; and decreasing kidney and bladder function.

As a result of relaxation, the physiological process of stress subsides. Noticeable changes are the alteration in the rate of breathing, blood pressure and the heartbeat lowering.

All forms of relaxation aim to help the patient to relax by reducing muscle tension and focusing their attention on something else to help alleviate their pain or stress.

Pain induces stress which in turn stimulates the autonomic nervous system into action which increases the respiratory rate, muscle tension and heart rate, which in turn can produce pain and therefore a vicious cycle which is difficult to break. By the introduction of relaxation you are hopefully going to have an effect in reducing the activity of the autonomic nervous system, thus reducing respiratory rate, heart rate and muscle tension.

The aim of relaxation is to reduce tension and restore the body's equilibrium. This can be achieved by teaching patients the difference between tense and relaxed positions and body state. This is done by a series of exercises based on a combination of the Mitchell method of physiological relaxation and the Jacobson method. This progressive muscle relaxation involves a methodical conscious relaxation of all body areas in sequence. The patient is encouraged to contract the muscles in one part of the body at a time, then relax them back into a comfortable position and be aware of the positioning. Techniques can be tailored to the individual.

Controlled breathing is practised throughout if this is appropriate. Diaphragmatic breathing is more effective, promoting relaxation rather than tension.

The patient should be fully supported either in a sitting position or semi-reclining.

These exercises have produced good results in patients who have felt controlled by their pain previously. They have claimed to have felt a regaining of control and are aware that this is something they have achieved themselves.

Visualization is then combined with the relaxation aiming to allow the patient to drift through pleasant images, thus enhancing a state of mental peace.

It is necessary for all this to happen in a quiet environment with no interruptions.

At our hospice a group session of relaxation is conducted every afternoon. All day hospice patients are invited to join in, as are any inpatients from the unit plus family, friends, volunteers and staff. If any patient has problems coping with a group session a little time later in the day can be set aside for an individual session. Before starting the session it is decided which 'visual journey' should be taken that day.

At the commencement there is a series of body awareness exercises combined with breathing exercises as mentioned already. Where a patient with respiratory problems may find it difficult, if not distressing, to attempt breathing exercises, they are advised not to focus on the breathing but to concentrate on the conscious relaxation of the body. So as not to induce a state of anxiety in the rest of the group, such patients are told that, on their expiration breath, they should feel as if they are sinking deep into the chair or bed, so that they feel fully supported. They close their eyes if they wish and in this peaceful state listen to a story of a 'journey'. This is told in a calm, slow, gentle voice.

Various visual journeys have been devised based on suggestions from the patients themselves. These include country walks on a spring day, walking along a beach on a tropical island (one elderly patient at the end of this journey said he had imagined himself at Canvey Island – not quite what was envisaged!), a walk in the woods, the Lake District, water rides, horse and carriage rides, etc.

With all of the journeys patients are asked to imagine the scene being set, leaving regular pauses and quiet moments for them to employ their own imaginations and visualizing things special to them. Many recall memories conjured up by the scene set – a walk along the beach with a loved one, memories of holidays past, childhood memories, things they used to be able to do and enjoy.

The whole session takes about 10–15 minutes. The visualization is always completed by returning to the starting point by retracing the steps taken. During the narration there is a lot of positive feeling input describing the warmth of the sun, the freshness of the clear air, the smells surrounding us, the sights, feelings of well-being and strength and being relaxed, positive and in control.

The journey is finalized by imagining the scene – a beautiful sunset, a peaceful village green, etc. – for a few moments, then slowly and gently bringing the group back to the room by making them aware of themselves, aware of their toes, fingers, breathing, listening to the outside noises – the birds chirping, the fall of rain. Then slowly and when they are ready, opening their eyes and bringing themselves back to the room.

Sometimes at the end of the session patients have been known to go to sleep; they are left in this relaxed state for a short while, allowing them often to catch up on some much needed rest. They usually express feelings of having felt very relaxed and refreshed on awakening.

A tape recording of the journeys has been made and copies are available for patients to take home with them to use or for use on the unit if any patient is having problems relaxing.

Patients, family and staff seem to really enjoy and benefit from these sessions; it is especially beneficial as the relaxation is self-controlled.

Moetzinger and Dauber in *The Management of the Patient with Breast Cancer* (1982) stated, 'Relaxation and visualization may help patients to participate in their care, stay positive and ease their anxieties and depression'.

AROMATHERAPY

Aromatherapy is an art and a science using natural plant essences in treatment. These concentrated essences, mostly extracted by distillation, are from plants, flowers, trees and herbs and are the life force of the plant. Aromatherapy is a truly holistic and natural therapy and its origins go back 5000 years. It takes into account mind, body and spirit.

Each oil has many qualities and great potential for healing and can be used therapeutically to treat a wide variety of complaints, particularly in today's stress-ridden society. So many ills are caused by stress and by using this natural, holistic approach, many unpleasant symptoms can be relieved. Used alongside conventional medicine in the care of cancer patients, it can bring about feelings of calmness and relaxation and even well-being and often helps the individual to cope with the distress of their illness.

Some oils are stimulating and invigorating while others are calming and soporific. The aromatherapist chooses the oil(s) to suit the individual using a holistic approach. It is necessary in cancer cases to know some medical history in order to alleviate unpleasant symptoms and give most comfort and relief – a truly natural way to improve quality of life and give TLC (tender loving care).

The oils can be applied using massage techniques – massage must be the oldest medical treatment known as we all rub an ache or pain instinctively. The concentrated oils must be diluted for massage in a vegetable base oil, e.g. almond, sunflower, grapeseed, etc. Only very light pressure is used in massaging cancer patients but there are other uses for the essences as aroma is very important. The undiluted oil can be dropped onto a cotton wool swab for inhalation, two drops of essential oil, e.g. eucalyptus, in steaming hot water can relieve bronchial congestion or up to six drops of essential oil in a bath of warm water can be very comforting. The oils can also be used in pot pourri or diffusers.

When used in massage, the skin absorbs the oil allowing the capillary circulation to distribute its therapeutic properties throughout the body. Several essential oils act as natural balancers and are called adaptogens, e.g. lemon and peppermint can be stimulant or relaxant, so that the oil will respond to the body's needs. This apparent contradiction can be confusing until you realize they are natural balancers. Research is going on in Vladivostock (Russia) into this group of natural products amongst which are the root ginseng and the herb peppermint.

Tony Balacs, a pharmacologist and Scientific Editor of the *International Journal of Aromatherapy*, recently wrote in the journal of his findings on absorption of essential oils into the body (Balacs, 1992). Warmth of the oil, body and room temperature play a large part in the time of absorption, but smell also plays a significant role too. Modern research has confirmed the therapeutic properties of essential oils and investigation is ongoing. Peter Holmes (1992) wrote in the *International Journal of Aromatherapy* of his studies on lavender oil and considered it to be one of the top 'stress busters', a habit breaker and crisis smoother, one of the most versatile of all the essential oils.

In June 1992 the British Complementary Medicine Association was launched, bringing member therapies a step closer to medical status and respectability, which was cautiously welcomed by the British Medical Association. In time, it is hoped that all practitioners of aromatherapy will be registered. Complementing, cooperating and consulting are the aims of the Association. The Tisserand Institute in Hove, Sussex, founded in 1987 by Robert Tisserand, offers training courses in aromatherapy and seminars for interested people, e.g. nurses, physiotherapists, doctors, etc. Many other bodies throughout the country do the same.

At a seminar held in the Royal Masonic Hospital, London, in September 1992, Carol Horrigan, a registered nurse, tutor and aromatherapist, lectured on the use of complementary therapies in cancer care. She treats cancer patients at some London hospitals with essential oils and she gave accounts of positive results enjoyed by her patients. This made me more enthusiastic to use my knowledge to the benefit of the patients at the hospice where I work two days each week. Having a nursing background is a great advantage; once I have a mental picture of the patient's diagnosis and have introduced myself, I can decide what oils would be best to use if they would like to experience aromatherapy. Most people need a simple explanation and not many refuse the chance to try it, but the most satisfying result is obtained when a patient will show obvious positive improvement or relief of distressing symptoms such as nausea or sickness. Many patients look forward to another chance to receive this caring treatment and sometimes their family members receive aromatherapy privately after seeing the good results achieved by their loved ones.

A few years ago I retired from district nursing after 38 years in the nursing profession. I qualified as a massage therapist and became more and more convinced that the use of essential oils in massage increased its benefits. I have seen much improvement in the well-being of the people I have treated and at times with surprisingly quick results.

A 55 year old lady with breast cancer was attending a day hospice. For many months she had 'migraine' type headaches which dominated her waking day and ruined her sleep. These were not related to her cancer (except for being stress-provoked) as tests had been carried out. She was glad to have some aromatherapy in the hope of getting some relief so I gave her a back, neck and shoulder massage using lavender, geranium and frankincense. She enjoyed this experience very much and felt calm and relaxed and her headache had vanished. During my treatment of her I demonstrated the various pressure points on her face, head and neck to relieve her severe headaches and hopefully prevent them becoming a migraine attack. (Shiatsu or acupressure is a Oriental therapy, some of which I use when giving aromatherapy massage.) A few days later I met this lady again, who announced with a smile that her headaches were '80% gone'! Thanks to the wonderful power of the oils her quality of life was improved. Now her husband makes sure she has lavender oil available which she can use neat on her neck and temples if feeling agitated or unable to sleep.

The day hospice patients say how much better they sleep after their day with us and I feel that as much as the oils, their enjoyment of being cared for and made to feel special is at the root of this.

An 83 year old gentleman had prostate cancer with pelvic involvement. He enjoyed having his abdomen gently massaged with bergamot, lavender and marjoram. His feet and legs were often massaged too and he would wait eagerly for my next visit. During my time with him he would talk about his 82 year old wife and his sadness at leaving her, but his lovely smile and the obvious comfort he received made me happy to spend time with him.

A lady in her early 40s was admitted to the hospice in a terminal stage of her illness. She was very withdrawn and sad as her husband had just died. She seemed unable to communicate, she never complained and just curled up in the fetal position most of the time. I talked with her for a while and she admitted to me that she was nauseous and had bad headaches. At first she was reluctant to have aromatherapy but accepted a hand massage and a gentle massage round her neck and shoulders. I also put some peppermint oil on a tissue and tucked this into the top of her nightie, explaining the aroma of peppermint and lavender could help to dispel her nausea and headache. Twenty minutes later I returned to find her nausea and headache had gone and she felt much better. She accepted soup for lunch and then slept for quite a while.

Pure lavender on finger tips applied to pulse spots, e.g. wrists, temples, etc., can bring relief to an anxious person who does not want a massage.

So often during treatment the sick person will talk about their family, their fears and worries and this in itself is therapeutic. So often a patient will say how comforting it is to feel warm gentle hands touching them, making them feel special. I feel my role is an extension of the nurse's caring role and overlaps with other caring personnel, i.e. physiotherapist, relatives, etc. I like the relative to stay while I treat the patient so that, seeing what I do, they may like to do the same either at home or in the hospice. I sometimes make up oils for their use.

The following essential oils are most commonly used:

Lavender and camomile	Calming, analgesic, can be added to an emollient cream to use on dry areas of skin
Rosewood and bergamot	Uplifting to the psyche
Geranium and rose	Good for dry skin
Rosemary and lemon	Mentally refreshing
Frankincense, jasmine, rose and petitgrain	Euphoric oils which can be beneficial in relieving grief and sadness
Peppermint	For digestive upsets. Good for aches and pains too
Marjoram	Lowers high blood pressure, eases cramps, aids digestion. Calming to mind and body
Sandalwood	Uplifting, refreshing and relaxing. Antidepressant

All oils have many properties and can be used to treat a wide variety of conditions.

When working at the hospice the staff say how nice it is to be 'aware' that the aromatherapist is around, even though they cannot always see me!

REFLEXOLOGY

Reflexology is being used more widely now for treating terminally ill patients.

There is very little documented evidence of scientific trial results available at present, although there are various papers in the process of being written which should be made available in the near future. However, the Institute for Complementary Medicine did state that many practitioners had contacted them with informal reports of their successes in treating patients who are terminally ill.

Reflexology is a therapy that has been used on patients for over 5000 years in various parts of the world. Using specific thumb and finger techniques a compression massage is applied to relax points in the feet or hands. It is believed that by stimulating these reflex points, a reaction is caused in corresponding parts of the body.

Reflexology is considered a natural and drugless method of treatment. The aims of the treatments are to improve the nerve and blood supply, reduce stress and tension, alleviate discomfort and induce a feeling of relaxation, thus contributing greatly to the well-being of the terminally ill patient, especially if they have been confined to bed for some time.

The reflexologist hopes to restore the body's balance and it is claimed that this often gives some patients relief from their symptoms.

Reflexology is based on the body being divided into ten longitudinal zones, running from head to tip of toes. Each zone is related to the line going through the body, each containing a finger and a toe. There are also lateral zones, the most commonly used of which are the shoulder line, diaphragm line and the waistline.

It is believed that tenderness in a specific part of the foot or hand indicates congestion and inflammation of that zone. Applying alternating pressures to this area will affect the whole zone area from foot to head.

The foot can be mapped out to represent all the organs of the body.

Reflexology is said to be safe to be used on everyone.

Dobbs (1985) writes of her experiences in using reflexology for the treatment of terminally ill patients. She sees the needs of those patients as being to decrease pain, to be materially comforted and to be psychologically comforted. Some therapists have created their own special techniques for use with terminally ill patients. Monica Anthony, a member of the British Registry of Complementary Practitioners, a therapist and teacher, also uses a holistic foot massage where the reflexes are combined with healing techniques, involving an awareness of the subtle energy field surrounding and permeating the body. A very light touch can be extremely powerful and it is also possible to work with the hands slightly away from the body. This approach is especially suitable for people who have become extremely sensitive to the slightest touch and/or who are in pain.

It is claimed that the healing touch facilitates relaxation and a feeling of well-being which alleviates stress, depression and anxiety, restoring a sense of wholeness, hence the term 'holistic'.

Although we do not have a reflexologist practising at the hospice at the moment, the use of a very simple foot and hand massage (using the principles of reflexology) appears to have been beneficial to some very anxious patients.

This technique was used recently on a 37 year old woman with cancer of the breast with secondaries, who was in a very anxious and distressed state. She was convinced she was about to die at any moment. While talking to her I discovered that she had always enjoyed having her feet massaged, so I asked her permission to try some gentle foot and hand massages. This I did, combined with some visualization, having found out where her favourite places were. Although her anxiety did not totally subside, she certainly appeared to calm down, her breathing pattern changed and became more even and she was able to relax into the treatment. The physical contact and the fact that someone was doing something for her and with her helped to reduce her state of anxiety. This lady actually said that having someone touch her made her feel more able to cope and was soothing.

The same technique was used with a middle-aged man suffering from motor neurone disease, who gained relief if his feet were massaged.

A NURSE'S VIEWPOINT

As a nurse it has been very exciting to witness the development of complementary therapies within the health service and to be able to work within an environment which allows you to learn and develop complementary skills.

Many patients and their families are quite unaware of the forms of treatment available to them at the hospice. Not all have readily come forward into our care. Quite often our patients are referred by health care professionals within the community because they recognize that the main carer needs some respite from the 24-hour caring. We enhance the family unit as a whole and respect their decision for us to share in their care. The most difficult part of entering into hospice care is the first step over the threshold, but once it has been made we begin to work together to maintain some quality of life.

Whatever form of complementary therapy you choose it is important to remember you are sharing your patients' most precious commodity – their time. Patients often arrive in a very terminal condition and it may take a couple of days to complete your assessment of their needs and those of the family. Once this assessment has been made, you can discuss with them which forms of therapy you feel they may benefit from.

The first complementary therapy you offer, almost unconsciously, is counselling. The moment you sit down with someone and give them your time you are giving them an opportunity to offload their worries and fears. Often patients are aware of their incurable condition but shy away from speaking of it with their family for fear of upsetting them.

Being able to speak openly and freely about their condition and problems relating to it can promote a great sense of relief, which is one of the first steps towards relaxation. Perhaps enabling a patient to address their situation allows them to progress through the emotional stages. These are described by Dr Elisabeth Kübler-Ross, a physician at the University of Chicago, as denial, anger, bargaining, sadness and acceptance. We see patients at all these different stages. Families also benefit from having someone listen to their fears and worries and very gradually, when you feel the time is right, you can withdraw and allow the family as a whole to share special times together with the knowledge that you are at hand for support if needed.

William Shakespeare wrote, 'There is nothing good or bad, but thinking makes it so'. Our imagination is a very powerful thing. Instead of allowing our imagination to conjure up negative thoughts and feelings, it is possible to guide it to work for us and induce positive feelings. I was able to put this to use whilst on night duty. A gentleman in my care was very restless, unable to sleep for long periods and was becoming agitated. I sat with him and after ensuring there was nothing I could do or get for him, we lapsed into talking quietly together. This gentleman had been a sailor and had travelled widely. He told me of the countries he had seen and I in turn told him I had not travelled too widely but if he would like to close his eyes I would take him for a visual walk. We walked through sweetsmelling fields and I asked him to feel the warmth of the breeze on his skin. I described the scene and talked positive feelings. When we reached the edge of the field you could hear the sea. He visibly relaxed as the walk progressed. I was not sure at what point he fell asleep, but I was sure he slept for a good few hours and was aware of the quality of his sleep later on awakening.

Another colleague related a similar experience when he was working with a patient and his wife who was visiting. They both were very anxious and stressed. He used a similar technique and was able after a short while to leave them both fast asleep – one in bed and one in the chair.

Visualization can also be used as a fighting tool along with its relaxation power. A middle-aged lady was admitted to the hospice for two weeks' respite care, often saying 'I'm not ready for this'. She was a very houseproud lady and found it very frustrating not to be able to work around the house as she had done all her married life. This lady was very open about her diagnosis and was able to discuss her fears and hopes with staff and family. I asked if she would like to try guided imagery to try to alleviate some of her frustrations about the situation. She said she would. Having made sure she was resting comfortably, I asked her to imagine her cancer cells as dust or dirt and she was to clean it up with a bucket and mop. She was asked to think of working from the cancer site, working it away, down and out. She 'worked' for several minutes and I asked her then to imagine herself resting in the garden, relaxing after the effort, and when she was ready, to come back to the room. She rested in her chair for one hour. Later she told me the exercise had made her feel that she was 'doing something positive' with her situation.

By understanding the principles behind many of the complementary therapies, we as a team can use this knowledge to help patients to achieve some control and peace of mind, thus improving their quality of life. Often a patient has said how much something as simple as a relaxation session or a therapeutic massage has helped them to feel a bit more in control.

CONCLUSION

It is important when treating a terminally ill patient to try and involve the carers as much as they wish. Getting involved in the care gives them an opportunity to feel part of the hospice team, e.g. being shown by the aromatherapist a simple hand and foot massage which they can then give the patient when needed. It may help them to overcome some of their negative feelings of uselessness and in turn be therapeutic for them.

It must be very difficult for the family of the terminally ill person to come to terms with the inevitable outcome of their loved one's illness; they themselves will be going through a gamut of emotions – fear, anger and helplessness to name a few. Many may benefit from some individual time spent with them to help them to cope. Aromatherapy or relaxation can be beneficial. Joining in a relaxation session with family and other patients facilitates a shared experience to be cherished.

ACKOWLEDGEMENTS

Special thanks to Monica Anthony LRAM.

REFERENCES

Balacs, T. (1992) Dermal crossing. *International Journal of Aromatherapy*, **4**(2), 23–5.

Dobbs, B.Z. (1985) Alternative health approaches. Paper presented at the Nursing Mirror/Royal Marsden Hospital Advanced Nursing Practice Conference, London.

Downie, P. (ed.) (1984) *Cash's Textbook of General Medicine and Surgical Conditions for Physiotherapists*, Faber and Faber, London.

Holmes, P. (1992) Lavender oil – a study in contradictions. *International Journal of Aromatherapy*, **4**(2), 20–2.

Horrigan, C. (1991/2) Complementary cancer care. *Journal of Aromatherapy*, **3**(4), 15–17; **4**(1), 18–19; **4**(2), 28–9.

Melzack, R. and Wall, P. (1982) *The Challenge of Pain*, Penguin Education, Middlesex, p. 261.

Moerzinger, C.A. and Dauber, L.G. (1982) The Management of the patient with breast cancer. *Cancer Nursing*, **5**, 287–92.

FURTHER READING

Chaitow, L. (1992) *The Stress Protection Plan – How to Stay Healthy under Pressure*, Thorsons, London.

Cobb, S.C. (1984) Teaching relaxation techniques to cancer patients. *Cancer Nursing*, **April**, 157–61.

Davis, P. (1988) *Aromatherapy: An A–Z*, C.W. Daniel, Saffron Walden.

Gillanders, A. (1987) *Reflexology – Ancient Answers to Modern Ailments*, Jenny Lee Publishing Services, Essex.

Horn, S. (1986) *Relaxation*, Thorsons, Wellingborough.

Kung, K. and Kung, B. (1982) *The Complete Guide to Foot Reflexology*, Thorson Publishing Group, Wellingborough.

Maxwell Hudson, C. (1988) *The Complete Book of Massage*, Dorling Kindersley, London.

Readers Digest Family Guide to Alternative Medicine (1991) David and Charles, Newton Abbot.

Rowden, L. (1984) Techniques in patients with breast cancer. Relaxation and visualisation. *Nursing Times*, **18**(37), 42–4.

Tisserand, R. (1992) *The Art of Aromatherapy*, C.W. Daniel, Saffron Walden.

Worwood, V.A. (1990) *The Fragrant Pharmacy*, Macmillan, London.

Issues of bereavement

20

GRIEF AND LOSS

This book is about caring for the dying patient and the family: it is not about caring for the bereaved. So why have I, a bereavement social worker, been asked to contribute? Because the carer's involvement with the family does not necessarily end with the death and because loss, with all its tasks, effects and emotions, is present on both sides of an anticipated death.

'We begin life with loss' (Viorst, 1988) and from then until the day we die loss is a frequent, normal part of our lives. It is there in every change in our circumstances and in every choice we make. Most of these losses cause only mild emotional disequilibrium because:

- they are small and bring us gains that more than compensate;
- they are developments on a chosen course;
- we are ready for and now assent to them;
- they are stages in the life cycle to which we have become reconciled.

Until we experience a major bereavement we tend to think and behave as if things, people and relationships last forever, ignoring all the accumulating evidence in our lives that nothing is permanent. I remember, with embarrassment now, the amazement I felt when an old lady said after the death of a lifelong friend, 'Belle has given herself back to God, as I always knew she would'. She surely couldn't mean that! As I slowly realized she did mean it, so far was I from recognizing impermanence, her attitude elicited in me respect bordering on awe!

Not all the deceased are mourned or even missed and there is a unique sadness about funerals attended only by cemetery and funeral directors' staff. I think such funerals should not happen, that there should be someone present to acknowledge that this person lived and died, but not all marriages are happy, not every one is good and the term 'dear departed' is not appropriate to all the dead. It is advisable to approach those we think are experiencing loss not with assumptions but with questions. What is this person thinking? What feelings do they have? What does this death mean to them at this time?

Mr and Mrs W were frail over-80s. For over 50 years their lives had been devoted to the care of a mentally handicapped daughter, Mary. On the day Mary died they had a brief discussion about whether to say something and then stood hand in hand as Mr W said, 'Now we can go'. Mary's death meant for them that they had completed their life's work and they could now depart in peace. They had succeeded, they were triumphant, they had seen their Mary through to the end. In their view death was a friend to all three of them provided only that Mary died first.

My dictionary defines grief as 'deep or violent sorrow'. It is one of the raging emotions that wrack those that loss has plunged into an empty, pointless, unfamiliar world.

Even for people as ready for death as Mr and Mrs W, the words 'She's gone' change the world. Until that moment it is possible to maintain in a hidden corner of the mind the idea that 'miracles do happen' and 'where there's life there's hope' as life ebbs away and courage and love prompt the thought, though probably not the words, 'Because I love you I will let you go. Goodbye'.

THE PATIENT

The advance of disease brings some losses to the patient – speech, independence, control, mobility, energy, healthy appearance perhaps. Other losses accrue from interruptions of normal activity by illness and treatment: these may include loss of status, job, financial security, contraction of the social network and, if the patient has to be in hospital, loss of home, garden and pets. Daily habits are changed as the sick person surrenders former roles and becomes the one everybody else looks after, inefficient, incapable. Plans are unfulfilled, some tasks are started but will not be completed and choices decrease until there are none.

It is distressing to sit in an outpatient queue and see those whose disease is more advanced than your own, knowing that if all does not go well, you will become as ill as they are. What must it be like to have to stay day and night beside a person who is senselessly noisy? Or beside a patient who has hordes of visitors? What must it be like when you urgently need the district nurse or GP and know you have to wait alone because others also need their care? When a death occurs, is there a feeling of 'whose turn next?' and how is the answer arrived at.

The feelings patients have about each other may be strong and important to them, whether positive or negative. Each person is part of the environment of the other, provided by us! If everyone in the room or on the home carer's visiting list has lost much already through illness and is waiting to die, what does a death or a new patient coming into the group mean to them?

THE STAFF

What powerful people! They can tell you that you are getting better or worse and they know! They can preserve your dignity in many small ways or they can strip you of it. They can prevent pain, take it away, cause it. They can come when you need them or leave you in your need. They will attend to you when you die, when you are dead. Yes, they are powerful, so it's best to be careful!

Many of us all our adult lives are fiercely independent. We 'keep ourselves to ourselves' and wouldn't dream of asking anyone for anything. And then comes serious illness. We have to ask for help. If at that point we are treated with understanding, kindness and respect, our response is likely to be gratitude and trust that seems out of proportion to the help given. Sometimes the response is very strong and the fact that death is coming soon frees the patient from concern about the future of the relationship being established.

Being a carer is one role in a lifetime of many roles and we cannot be unaware that in time we will be in the place of the family and of the patient. For some this is one of the attractions of terminal care work – there is no us and them, just us. However, we should be attentive to the effect of continuous contact with dying, death and bereavement on ourselves and each other, especially when there is actual or threatened loss of life in professional carers' families.

We learn not to get too close to the dying in order to avoid grief. Yet the occasional patient slips below our guard. Perhaps the hardest part is not the empty bed but that so soon there is someone else in it. A carer may do much for and with a sick person, then have a couple of days off and find on their return that the patient died, another has come and so much has happened on the ward that no-one mentions the missing person at all. It is to be hoped that a carer who finds themselves troubled by circumstances like this will ask for information about the death and that their colleagues will recognize that there is unfinished business here they can help bring to completion.

For a professional to admit to strong feelings about a sick person is not easy and if those feelings are negative, it is almost impossible. Professor Michael Rothenberg led the way in 1967 when he drew attention to the conflict in those caring for dying children caused by 'two powerful and normal but antithetical emotional responses elicited by the patients': the response of compassion causing movement towards the child with help and the response of repulsion in order to protect oneself from failure and loss, causing movement away.

> Our resolution must come from consciously forcing ourselves toward the patient and his family, while simultaneously recognizing, expressing and finally, understanding and thus coping with the many reactions that would trigger off our movement in the opposite direction.
> (Rothenberg, 1974)

Dr Robert Twycross (1990) has shown us another conflict.

> I would like to say two things which I hope will show that I am neither unfeeling nor uncaring. First, a doctor who has never been tempted to kill a patient has probably had very limited clinical experience or is not able to empathize clearly with those who suffer: second, the doctor who leaves a patient to suffer intolerably is morally more reprehensible than the doctor who opts for 'death assistance'.

Dr Sheila Cassidy (1988) wrote:

> There comes a time when the carers' hands are empty, when all the treatment manoeuvres have been explored, all the words of comfort said. It is then that one is left standing at the foot of the bed, useless, impotent, wanting more than anything else to run away.

Jean Vanier (1990) left the leadership of L'Arche to live in a community with four deeply handicapped persons. One of them, Lucien, could not speak, but screamed often.

> Something happened inside me when he started this screaming. The depths of his anguish triggered off my anguish, too. There was nothing we could do when he went into these fits, no way of reaching him in his pain and touching him in love. So I saw rising up inside myself incredible anguish and fear, close even to hate, and I saw in myself that I had the capacity to hurt.

We cannot avoid such feelings without blunting our sensitivity, but we can learn to deal with them so that they neither deter us from our chosen caring role or leave a residue of destructive guilt.

FAMILY AND FRIENDS

Hospital, hospice and home nurses, home helps, social workers and neighbours, we all see the relatives and friends arrive with flowers and titbits of food and clean laundry and we all help patients be ready to greet them. We see the greeting and how they arrange themselves around the patient. It is rather like reading the last page of a novel or a biography without having read any of the earlier pages. So again we must make no assumptions but keep questions in our mind.

It is hard when illness strikes and life is threatened to cope with the knowledge that your death will cause anguish to your nearest and dearest, that the people you most want not to hurt will be hurt, that those you would most like to comfort in their times of grief will feel your absence very keenly. In my view, for some people, this is the sting in the tail of life, not dying or death.

The feelings underlying the question 'How will they manage without me?' are complex, strong and painful. The answer is, of course, 'I don't know', but said as one settles down and prepares to listen to both the patient and the person they are concerned for. Maybe, carer and patient working together can build the courage of the person soon to be bereaved, removing the sting in the tail of life for the patient and making the bereavement more endurable.

Decades of increasing life expectancy have led to many more people living through their 60s and 70s to die in late old age, when their children are already elderly. Care of the frail old dying or bereaved person may fall heavily on someone unable or unwilling to meet the demands. Mrs M's niece complained bitterly that she had done her best for her aunt but she had not been able to do as much as Mrs M's children thought she should. There were three of them. They all lived more than 50 miles away from her: one of them had no car, one had severe heart trouble and the third had cancer. The niece lived near to Mrs M and was prepared to spend two hours twice a week helping her. Mrs M's needs grew and so did the time and energy the niece gave her until she felt she had no time for herself, her husband, her children and still she could not meet the needs of her aunt or the hopes of Mrs M's children.

The family and friends are waiting and whether they wait for the death, the recovery or to see what will happen, normal life is postponed for them. What will they be doing next week? That depends . . . Something very important is happening over which they have no control.

> I want to stay awake: I'd hate to be asleep when daddy dies, but I've stayed awake four nights now . . .
>
> Die. Just die. I can't go on like this.
>
> I don't know whether to pray she lives or pray she dies. Is that wicked of me?
>
> I feel so helpless.
>
> I can't bear to see her like this but I can't bear to be away from her either.

> I went to the window to see if there was anyone I could call to help. There was no-one there. He died while I was looking for help . . .

These statements were made by six bereaved people reliving earlier events. None of them is unusual. They are written to remind us of the range of feelings the person sitting at the bedside may be experiencing. Some sit and wait for the death to happen. Others sit and hope it won't, that the patient will 'turn the corner'. Some are bored and may be guilty about that. If the dying person appears to be in pain or distress, emotion in the person keeping vigil may boil up and find expression in words or actions.

Relationships and duties not concerned with the patient are shelved and some face the question 'How long can I be away from work and still pay the mortgage and keep my job?'. Other members of the family may be deprived of their normal quota of attention and come to resent the sick person: if a dying parent is well attended by her daughter, how do that daughter's husband and children fare? And does she feel torn in two by these conflicting demands? Even simple routine personal matters can cause conflict – do you leave the bedside to eat, shop, bath, sleep or do you wait in case the patient wakes up and wants you or dies?

A patient dies. A nurse says, 'She's gone'. For some, that is the moment at which the loss occurs. Others speak of learning the diagnosis or other episodes during the illness as being the time they sustained their loss. Mrs A lost her husband as he jumped up from the dining room table to leave hand marks on the ceiling. That day he was sectioned and a month later brain cancer was diagnosed. As he was dying some months later she was unmoved – her problem was not that her husband was dying but that she couldn't yet bury the person she lost months before.

Mrs O illustrates the opposite end of the spectrum. She could not hear, could not believe that her husband had cancer. He had flu, she said. When he died, her three children, all in their 30s, arranged the funeral. She attended dressed in black but not at all distressed. To someone who spoke conventional words of condolence, she said in apparent amusement, 'Oh no! It's not Bert's funeral! He only had flu!'. About the children's wreaths, she said, 'Look – three people with the same names as you three have lost their dad'. It was another ten weeks before she allowed herself to realize her husband had died and a lot longer before she could believe he had not had flu, but cancer.

For Mrs A, the nurse's words 'He's gone' were external ratification of something she had known for a long time, regardless of any evidence to the contrary. To Mrs O, that moment did not take place until she was ready to admit that the unthinkable had happened. Such cases are rare, though it is not rare to hold on to the past circumstances and delay the unknown future by an hour or two, or a day or two, through shock, numbness, denial or conscious choice.

It is not unusual to meet people at sickbeds and funerals that you have not seen for many years, if ever. Families and friends gather whether or not they know each other or like each other. I recall one patient in the middle of one wife, two ex-wives and the adult children of all three marriages. None of them had expected to be confronted by the other visitors and it was an uncomfortable experience for everyone.

The gay partner is now likely to be accepted by ward staff as next of kin until the patient's mother arrives: similarly, the common law wife is likely to be accepted until the patient's son arrives. Then the gay partner and common law wife may find they have no right to information, possessions or even notification. One common law wife had lived with her partner for seven years, disapproved of by his two sons whose mother had died when they were in their 20s. They, of course, were next of kin and they held the funeral without telling her the arrangements so she could not attend. One can sympathize with them – they buried their father with their mother, uniting the family, but in so doing they excluded the woman who felt herself to be the widow and complicated her bereavement.

If the patient wishes to protect his common law wife and ensure she has the legal rights and state benefits due to a widow, marriage is an option! It can be arranged and held in a few days with the cooperation of the Registrar if both partners are free to marry, wish to do so, are mentally clear and one of them is close to death. There is another way. As a Lighthouse leaflet states:

> It is especially important to make a will if you are gay or unmarried and have a partner you wish to provide for. If you do not make a will, your partner has no legal right to look after your affairs or to inherit anything of yours.

The question we have to ask, then, is 'Is there a will?' and if so, 'Who is the executor?'. That is the person with the right to information, notification and the possessions, though it is to be hoped the executor will agree to a free flow of communication to all concerned with the patient.

It usually happens that by common consent one of the family is designated chief mourner and the rest delay, hide or withhold any grief they may have in order to support that person. The widow is usually assigned chief mourner role while the sons and daughters assist her.

Problems arise for carers when no common consent is possible. When Mr D died his family consisted of four children aged 17 to 23. None of them was present at the death though all had previously visited him and all were expected shortly. There was anxiety among the staff. They did not want any of the children to walk in and find dad dead in bed and neither did they want them to walk in and find an empty bed, but how much time could they give to watching the ward entrance? As the children arrived, the problems for the staff grew worse because all four reacted strongly but in totally different ways: one got started at once on phoning relatives, one screamed and cried, one became silent and motionless and one, the only boy in the group, paced the room angrily shouting 'I'm sorry, dad'. What was the senior nurse to do with all of them? What she did was to ask for immediate help. The chaplain came at once and was asked to give his attention to the boy: they went off together to talk to dad. The social worker came at once and took the screaming, crying youngster to a more private room close by. The senior nurse herself took the one who was phoning relatives to the ward office so she could facilitate and monitor progress. The one who became silent and motionless stayed still where she was, an auxiliary with her trying to get her to drink tea until her sister returned from phoning.

The troubles of the patient will soon be over but we know that even if the survivors feel relief, they have difficult months or years ahead of them. There are things you can do for the dying, but what can you do for those left? So it is that terminal carers may find dealing with the relatives is the most painful part of their work.

For all of us, patient, relative and carer, there is a time to fight and a time to give in, a time to hold on and a time to let go. As professionals we must be able and willing to accept what each person's inner clock is telling them and then strive to harmonize, synchronize the timings within the family. Mrs F was not ready to let her husband go when the GP 'said to me, very slowly he said it, "Mary, Joe wants to go. Joe **wants** to go." '. Joe died some months after that and Mary was ready, prepared by those few words.

OTHER PATIENTS

At events for the bereaved there is sometimes evident pleasure as widows who last met while visiting their husbands greet each other with warmth and concern. Some continue to visit the ward, maintaining relationships made with other patients until there is no-one left from the days when their relative was there. In the time that one is awaiting a death few words have to be said, if any, for all those present in mind and body to understand the situation and identification can then be a powerful aid in pregrief work.

Mrs B sat two feet away from her husband's bed, ramrod stiff, erect, unmoving. This was her second husband: the first had died 20 years previously and soon after, her only son had attempted suicide. A nurse came, screened the bed, and she had to leave while the nurse attended to the patient. As she emerged from behind the screens Alf in the bed opposite held his arms out to her. She went to him, bent her ramrod back and accepted his hug. 'He'll be better off dead, mate,' Alf murmured and she cried in his arms. When she returned to her husband's bed she was able to sit closer and take his hand. Alf had achieved far more for her than I could.

THE CAREGIVERS

You come with your friend or relative to this big, busy place and are led into a ward, to a bed and there you are separated. You are in a strange world, home to others but not to you. Anxiety mounts: what is happening to the patient and what is expected, even demanded, of you? What are the rules you should obey? Are they the same as the other hospitals in the earlier stages of the illness? Some struggle with the fear that they might 'disgrace' themselves by showing emotion of any sort in front of the professional carers. Some see themselves as useless and helpless in contrast with the skilled staff now tending the sick person. For some there is guilt, especially if the patient wished to die at home.

Ward routines and doctors' and nurses' visits may interrupt or disturb the patient; this can lead to irritation and the angry question who do they belong to anyway?

Like the patients, relatives have good cause to see the professional carers as powerful people it is not safe to displease and even to ask a question may feel risky. To believe that the nurses are angels is very comfortable. The relative can leave the bed and go away trusting that their patient is in safe hands, getting the best possible care, better even than they could give. Guilt about not having the patient at home or not being able to make them comfortable at home is assuaged. They have not been abandoned for selfish reasons but entrusted to superior beings for selfless ones.

The vulnerability of their position makes it difficult for relatives and friends of the dying to see facts and events dispassionately. Three years after Mrs P's husband died she talked of incidents on the day he was transferred to a hospice from a general hospital. He had been sitting in a chair, sliding forward on the shiny seat, and she had asked that he be placed on his bed to await the ambulance in greater comfort. Her request was refused. 'Why wouldn't she do it?' she said repeatedly. It wasn't a question – she was not seeking an answer. Her anger mounted and raged. 'Hitler wasn't as cruel as that woman! She's not fit to nurse! She's not fit to live!' Her inability to help Mr P at that time, guilt from feeling she was betraying him in his hour of need and that they were both being betrayed by all health professionals made it impossible for her to be rational.

CARE OF THE BEREAVED

In the first few weeks there is much to be done: suddenly 'the law' is interested in the deceased and their possessions in the form of coroners and income tax officials, perhaps the police, pension and insurance offices, housing benefit, building society and bank staff, solicitors, funeral directors, the Registrar and even the High Court. There is a funeral to be arranged and the social event that precedes or follows it, according to custom. There is a gathering of the clan, not all of whom are known and not all of whom are acceptable to the bereaved. There is likely to be a full address book: 'Every time I told someone, I ended up comforting them' said one widow. She also found that every time she told someone, she believed it a little more herself.

If the bereaved is a member of a small, cohesive subculture group, it is likely there will be a clear prescript to be followed and although the bereaved person has lost much, that loss is shared and a sense of belonging remains. Most in our inner cities and dormitory countryside are not so fortunate. Mrs J lives in a slim tower block where no-one ever passes her door. This doesn't trouble her – she and her husband kept themselves to themselves and didn't socialize with anyone. They had one child, a daughter, who hasn't darkened their door since her stormy adolescence. Three years ago Mrs J's husband died and she is still enfolded in grief. In most weeks she speaks three times, once to the milkman when she pays her bill, once to the supermarket checkout person and once to her sister-in-law who comes ten miles to visit her weekly despite her own serious ill health. 'My brother in New Zealand would like me to go and join him, but I can't do that,' she says plaintively. She and her husband lived in a world of two and two minus one doesn't leave one, it leaves an empty world.

The busyness of the first few weeks and the support given in that period come to an end. No more visits to the hospital. No more clinic appointments. No more nurses visiting. No more favourite meals to tempt. No more thank you letters to write. No-one to look after, no-one to care. 'I was first in his life,' said one widow, 'and I'll never be first to anyone again.' During the months to come those left discover slowly what they have lost and painfully adjust to their new situation.

William Worden wrote:

> I don't believe we need to establish a new profession of grief counsellors. D.M. Reilly, a social worker, says 'We do not necessarily need a whole new profession of . . . bereavement counsellors. We do need more thought, sensitivity and activity concerning this issue on the part of existing professional groups; that is clergy, funeral directors, family therapists, nurses, social workers and physicians.' I couldn't agree more.

The professional most likely to be part of a bereaved person's support network is the GP. Two major reasons for this are: 'Bereaved people often report that their 'general health' has been worse following bereavement; they tend to consult doctors more frequently than non-bereaved controls and to report a higher prevalence of the symptoms of ill health' (Parkes and Weiss, 1983). Christina Victor (1993), using the Mortality Statistics of the Office of Population Censuses and Surveys, has shown that there has been a significant demographic change in the age at which death occurs in just 18 years. In 1969, 40% of those who died were 75 or over. In 1987, 55% were over 75.

> Increasing life expectancy means that people dying in 1987 had a rather different set of problems from the dying in 1969. Physically, they were in greater need, and having fewer family members around them to support them there was more dependence on formal services for help.

Increasing life expectancy also means that bereavement comes to those ever more old and frail.

Some of the bereaved will go to the doctor just because that's the person to whom you take your pain. Others will seek help from the clergy or spiritualists because they know about the hereafter. A few will need to be referred to specialists, psychiatrists or grief therapists. Some will move, to live with a relative or go into residential care perhaps. Most will come through the dark tunnel in the strength of their own capacity to survive with the help of neighbours, friends and relatives.

In recent years many organizations have come into being to support the bereaved. All offer the opportunity to talk and to be listened to, usually through home visits by trained volunteers, though some also provide group meetings, telephone helplines or office interviews. Many also offer one or more of the following:

- a legal and financial advice service;
- social events;
- rituals of remembrance;
- relevant cards, leaflets, books;
- information about local resources (e.g. what child care facilities are there to help the father of young children hoping to get back to work after the death of his wife?).

Local organizations for the bereaved are not easy to locate and of course they do not exist everywhere. Reference libraries, citizens advice bureaux, social service departments, volunteer bureaux, hospital social workers and hospices can all be expected to know of those in their area and the National Association of Bereavement Services (see Useful Addresses), is there to help with just this question.

'We must never be too sure we know what is best or most appropriate for others in dealing with their grief.' This applies to all bereavement work, but particularly so in the context in which Monica McGoldrick

(Walsh and McGoldrick, 1991) wrote it – mourning in different cultures. Our culture gives us assumptions that determine to a large degree our ideas, emotions and behaviour, our expectations, values, language and relationships and motivations. To illustrate this, a white Anglo-Saxon Protestant teacher asked a racially mixed adolescent girls class whether doctors should end the life of a seriously deformed baby. 'Would it be better for the baby or not,' she asked. 'It depends on whose fault it was he was born that way,' came the first answer. 'If it was his fault, then he would just be reborn the same. If it was his parent's fault, then it would be better for him.' This answer was totally unexpected by the teacher, 'blinkered' by her own culture. A second example comes from my own bereavement work. I visited a Muslim man soon after the death of his wife. It did not occur to me that he might not be the person most bereaved by his wife's death: he had visited her regularly in hospital and spent long hours with her in her last days, which no-one else had. In fact much the greatest loss had been sustained by his second wife: he had seen little of either of them, but they had been inseparably linked. When I visited him I didn't know of her existence and didn't even wonder if he had a second wife.

McGoldrick suggests that to understand a cultural group's traditions we need to discover:

- what the prescribed rituals are concerning dying, death and bereavement;
- what beliefs are held about the future, if any, of the dead;
- what they believe about appropriate emotional expression and integration of a loss experience;
- what the gender rules are for the bereaved;
- whether certain deaths are stigmatized within the group or particularly traumatic for them.

However, this is only a beginning of the learning necessary if we are to be effective bereavement workers for people of a culture other than our own and if the day should ever come when we have all the knowledge we need about every culture and subculture in our multiracial inner cities, we may still, in areas of high immigration, have a problem being sensitive enough and intuitive enough to understand a person speaking at best in their second language and at worst through an interpreter.

What is this person thinking? What feelings do they have? What have they lost? We must make no assumptions; we do not know until the bereaved person tells us and explains and even then we know only for that moment – five minutes later they may be thinking something different, feeling another emotion, discovering another loss. In talking and in our understanding, the journey towards letting go both of the deceased and of the grief moves forward.

BEREAVED CHILDREN

When children are bereaved, like adults they must complete tasks of mourning before they can move forward in their lives with hope and expectation for the future. Sadly, however, many adults are afraid of helping children complete these tasks in a mistaken belief that they are protecting the child. In reality, they are in fact trying to protect themselves.

Susan Bach, a Jungian analyst, has studied the spontaneous drawings of terminally ill children which can reveal their knowledge of not only their own impending death but the purpose of their illness and brief life and future life after death (Kübler-Ross, 1982, pp. 17–18, 66–7).

Many people in Western society perceive death as an unpleasant fact of life and think children should be shielded from such an event, but children need to experience the pain and grief of loss and be included in the mourning rituals of adult society such as the cremation or funeral, sharing the grief whether it be within the family, school or community.

The concept of death develops gradually in childhood and by the age of six many children are beginning to appreciate that death is forever. Adults should use concrete language when speaking with a bereaved child, using such words as 'dead', allowing the child, if possible, to feel the dead person as part of saying 'goodbye', perhaps feeling for a pulse or holding a mirror against the mouth to prove that the person is no longer alive.

The thinking of children, particularly those under seven, is very much dominated by visual impressions and reality and truth are more likely to help a child reach some understanding of events as opposed to distortion or evasion of facts.

Literature provides us with some excellent examples of children's intuitive and cognitive ability to grasp facts and discern whether or not they are being told the truth. In Charles Dickens' *Dombey and Son*, the six year old Florence goes to her little brother's wet nurse to find out where her mother has gone.

Florence says, 'What have they done with my Mama?'

The nurse does not reply directly but tries to divert Florence by asking her a question.

'My darling,' says Richards, 'you wear that pretty black frock in remembrance of your Mama?'

'I can remember my Mama,' returned the child, with tears springing to her eyes, 'in my frock.'

'But people put on black, to remember people when they're gone.'

'Where gone?' ask the child.

'Come and sit down by me,' said Richards 'and I'll tell you a story.'

Florence quickly perceived that she will get her answers to questions about her mother's death and listens to what the nurse has to say.

Mrs Richards uses concrete language, saying 'she was buried in the ground where the trees grow'. To the child the ground is a cold place but the nurse explains very beautifully how lovely flowers grow out of the ground and, choosing words that enable the child to use her imagination creatively to provide her with answers and some comfort, she assures her it is all right to feel sad and cry, at the same time physically comforting the child.

A lovely illustration often used by those who work with bereaved and dying children is the analogy of the body being like a chrysalis after the butterfly has flown free and Elisabeth Kübler-Ross (1978) describes seeing drawings of butterflies on the walls of the Maidanek concentration camp in Poland amongst messages to mothers and fathers.

Children react to bereavement very much like adults. Denial and anger may manifest themselves by regression, sadness, anger towards others, educational difficulties, hopelessness and despair, disbelief, preoccupation and confusion. A child needs to be reassured that these feelings are not peculiar to them alone. They are normal feelings most adults and children experience after they lose someone they love.

A child may show acceptance of loss by a direct statement, 'My brother is dead, he is not coming back here' or by asking to move to a dead sibling's bedroom or retain specific possessions. These personal effects provide for a child comfort and a sense of continuity, the sorting out process helping them to reinvest their emotional energy.

Dr Bluebond Langer (1978) talks about respecting the defence mechanisms. Children aged between six and nine may admit unhappiness but children between nine and 12 rarely do.

A desire to continue normal activities such as school should be respected. One young teenage boy known to the writer returned to school the day after his young brother's death from a medical condition affecting them both. He was quite realistic but to stay at home with a household of grieving relatives including his mother was more than he could cope with. He knew both the school staff and his peer group would understand and be supportive. Only by taking this course of action could he begin to accept the inevitability of his own death in the not too distant future.

Bereavement may change a child's status in the family. Perhaps they are now the eldest or youngest family member, perhaps they feel responsible for the parent left behind and it is not uncommon for an older child to want to feel involved in household decision making. It is important that the child's concerns are treated with respect. They may have to take on responsibilities more appropriate to an older person but the future adult is likely to have extra qualities of compassion and understanding in their approach to life.

Adults can help children come to terms with the reality of loss by working together on a memory book. One school class of young children made such a book to send to a deceased pupil's mother. Needless to say it had pride of place in the family home. Anniversaries, too, are very important occasions and should be made special, doing things that the bereaved person would have enjoyed. Children need to be reassured that it is in order for them to enjoy themselves and laugh.

Children and young people with learning difficulties may still, even today, be expected to cope with not only a bereavement but immediate drastic changes in their lifestyle such as going into residential care and living with people previously unknown to them. Sometimes they may not even be told about the death of the parent because it is assumed that they will be either too upset or unable to understand. Even if a child is so disabled as to seem unaware of a caring parent or know them as 'mum' or 'dad', great thought needs to be given towards helping them understand that the beloved carer is no longer there. Physical comfort, preferably from a known person, is vital, as is allowing the child to feel specific possessions such as clothing and telling them what has happened even if they would not appear to understand. Continuing routines and minimizing carers is very important, trying to allow only those who have always known the child or young person to care for them, particularly over intimate care details.

People with learning difficulties grieve just the same as those with greater intellectual ability and need similar support to help them readjust to a changed environment.

As noted at the beginning of this section, the process of grieving often begins long before the actual death of the loved one. Where death of a parent or sibling is anticipated and not sudden, the child will find their whole world altered in a bewildering and disturbing way, whether the dying relative is at home or in hospital or hospice. They need special attention and warm affection from an adult who will help the child understand the situation as their age and temperament allow. Hopefully, this can be within the family circle and many hospices encourage the whole family to meet together to talk with a counsellor about this important time in all their lives. Sometimes children are helped also by being invited to express their feelings through drawing when they are unable to do so orally. It is crucial that the child is not shut out from the unfolding events by a well-meaning conspiracy of evasion and actual physical exclusion from the parent, brother or sister who is dying.

After the death of a loved one we should move forward in our lives, taking with us the lessons learnt through the tasks of mourning. To deny these lessons to any child may have long-lasting effects from which they may never fully recover.

REFERENCES

Bluebond-Langner, M. (1978) *The Private Worlds of Dying Children*, Princeton Press, New Jersey.

Cassidy, S. (1988) *Sharing the Darkness*, Darton, Longman and Todd, London, p. 58.

Dickens, C. (1848) *Dombey and Son*, Penguin Classics, London.

Kübler-Ross, E. (1978) *To Live Until We Say Goodbye*, Prentice Hall, New Jersey.

Kübler-Ross, E. (1982) *Living with Death and Dying*, Souvenir Press, London.

Parkes, C.M. and Weiss, R. (1983) *Recovery from Bereavement*, Basic Books, New York.

Rothenberg, M. (1974) Problems posed for staff who care for the child, in *Care of the Child Facing Death*, (ed. L. Burton), Routledge and Kegan Paul, London, p. 39.

Twycross, R. (1990) Assisted death: a reply. *Lancet*, **336**, 796–8.

Vanier, J. (1990) Life with the poor; life from the poor. *Tablet*, **244**, 16–17.

Victor, C. (1993) Health policy and services for dying people and their carers, in *Death, Dying and Bereavement*, (eds D. Dickenson and M. Johnson), Sage Publications, Milton Keynes.

Viorst, J. (1988) *Necessary Losses*, Simon and Schuster, London.

Walsh, F. and McGoldrick, M. (1991) *Living Beyond Loss: Death in the Family*, W.W. Norton and Co., New York.

Worden W. (1991) *Grief Counselling and Grief Therapy*, 2nd edn, Routledge, London.

FURTHER READING

Arranging Your Affairs and Making a Will, Terrence Higgins Trust leaflet, London.

Dyregron, A. (1990) *Grief in Children – A Handbook for Adults*, Jessica Kingsley, London.

Grollman, E.A. (ed.) (1969) *Explaining Death to Children*, Beacon Press, Boston.

Hurst, S. (1977) *Shaken by the Wind*, Mayhew-McCrimmon, Great Wakering.

Krementz, J. (1983) *How It Feels When a Parent Dies*, Victor Gollancz (also helpful for children to read).

Seale, C.F. (1993) Demographic change and the care of the dying, in *Death, Dying and Bereavement*, (eds D. Dickenson and M. Johnson), Sage Publications, Milton Keynes.

For children

Heegaard, M.E. (1988) *When Someone Very Special Dies*, Woodland Press, New York.

Stickney, D. (1982) *Water Bugs and Dragonflies – Explaining Death to Children*, Mowbray, London.

Useful addresses

Association of Chartered Physiotherapists in Oncology and Palliative Care
St Catherine's Hospice, 137 Scalby Road, Scarborough YO12 6TB
Tel. 0723 351421

Association of Hospice Social Workers
East Cheshire Hospice, Millbank Drive, Macclesfield SK10 3DR
Tel. 0625 610364

Association of Hospice Voluntary Services Coordinators
St Leonard's Hospice, 185 Tadcaster Road, York YO2 2QL
Tel. 0904 708553

BACUP (Information and Support Service for Cancer Sufferers)
3 Bath Place, Rivington Street, London EC2A 3JR
Tel. 071 613 2121

Cancer Relief Macmillan Fund
15/19 Britten Street, London SW3 3TZ
Tel. 071 351 7811

Compassionate Friends
53 North Street, Bedminster, Bristol BS3 1EN
Tel. 0272 539639

CRUSE, National Organization for the Widowed and Their Children
CRUSE House, 126 Sheen Road, Richmond, Surrey TW9 1UR
Tel. 081 940 4818

Marie Curie Cancer Care
28 Belgrave Square, London SW1X 8QG
Tel. 071 235 3325

Help the Hospices
34–44 Britannia Street, London WC1X 9JG
Tel. 071 278 5668

Hospice Information Service
St Christopher's Hospice, 51–59 Lawrie Park Road, London SE26 6DZ
Tel. 081 778 9252

Lesbian and Gay Bereavement Project
Vaughan M. Williams Centre, Colindale Hospital, London NW9 5HG
Tel. 081 200 0511 (a recording giving the name and number of the person on call is obtainable on 081 455 8894)

National Association of Bereavement Services
20 Norton Folgate, London E1 6DB
Tel. 071 247 0617

National Association of Funeral Directors
57 Doughty Street, London WC1
Tel. 071 242 9388

National Association of Hospice/Palliative Day Care Leaders
Sir Michael Sobell House, Mount Vernon Hospital, Rickmansworth Road, Northwood, Middx HA6 2RY
Tel. 0895 278302

Stillbirth and Neonatal Death Society
28 Portland Place, London W1N 4DE
Tel. 071 436 5881

The Terrence Higgins Trust
52–54 Gray's Inn Road, London WC1X 8JU
Tel. 071 242 1010

Religious bodies

Association of Hospice Chaplains
Strathcarron Hospice, Randolph Hill, Denny, Stirling, Scotland FK6 5HJ
Tel. 0304 826222

Buddhist Hospice Trust
P.O. Box 123, Ashford, Kent TN24 9TF
Tel. 081 789 6170

Hospital Chaplains' Fellowship
c/o Reverend David H. Robinson, Wallsgrave Hospital, Clifford Bridge Road, Wallsgrave, Coventry, West Midlands CV 2DX
Tel. 0203 613232

Islamic Cultural Centre
146 Park Road, London NW8 7RG
Tel. 081 724 3363

Jewish Joint Burial Society
North-Western Reform Synagogue, Alyth Gardens, London NW11 7EN
Tel. 081 455 8579

United Synagogue (Orthodox)
Woburn House, Upper Woburn Place, London WC1H OE7
Tel. 071 387 4300

Index